THE SPIRULINA COOKBOOK

Recipes for Rejuvenating the Body

Sonia Beasley

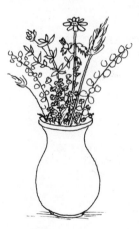

University of the Trees Press   P.O. Box 644   Boulder Creek, CA 95006

Printed in the United States by R.R. Donnelley & Sons Company.

LIBRARY OF CONGRESS CATALOGING IN PUBLICATION DATA

Beasley, Sonia, 1941—
   The Spirulina cookbook.

   Includes index.
   1. Marine algae as food.   2. Cookery (Spirulina)
I. Title.
TX402.B4   641.6   81-40027
ISBN 0-916438-39-2 (pbk.)   AACR2

ACKNOWLEDGEMENTS

My deepest respect and gratitude goes to the late Dr. Hiroshi Nakamura,
who, over the last three decades pioneered the research into Spirulina
as a world future food with dedication and conviction. And to Dr.
Christopher Hills, who pioneered with Dr. Nakamura and who is making
this wonderful super food available to the world. And to the staff of the
book production department of University of the Trees Press for their
fine work in designing, editing, typesetting and pasting up this book.

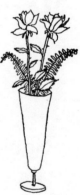

Illustrations by Reenie Haughey

CONTENTS

BACKGROUND

I have asked Sonia Beasley to publish these recipes for making Spirulina dishes because she has tested them all out on the students at the University of the Trees for some time and received feedback on their practicality and tastiness so that just the right amount of Spirulina can be used without affecting the normal palette.

Of course there are those people, like my wife Norah, who just love the marine taste of kelp and just love the seaweed taste of Spirulina so much that they suck the tablets all day long. Others can't take the powder in the mouth right away and they prefer to swallow Spirulina in tablet form. However, I have noted that once the body gets to like the tablets then those who didn't like its taste at first become converts after a month and start taking the powder in soups, smoothies, and eventually finish up chewing the tablets like my wife. So an initial reaction on the tongue is not to be taken as the body's final answer.

Everyday I get letters and most days telephone calls from grateful people who have been so pleased with the effects of Spirulina on their bodies that it amazes me how easily Spirulina sells itself. It even turns skeptics into believers without any words once they begin to use it for fasting or for losing weight.

Obviously we are not allowed to make any therapeutic claims for it because of FDA regulations, but we can say that in other countries, notably in Mexico and Japan the government equivalents of the FDA have tested it and found it absolutely safe for babies and adults and for use by doctors in the treatment of various diseases, in those countries. Whether the FDA will approve it for more than a food supplement we cannot say, but what we can say is that many people have used it solely as a dietary supplement and have subsequently found it to have a fantastic effect on their health. We have hundreds of unsolicited testimonials from people who have suffered for years who have written us to say that their problems have gone away. One day we may publish these letters once we know it is safe to do so without the FDA accusing us of recommending it for medical problems. We advise all users not to make extravagant claims concerning its effects on disease and instead talk about its effects on health. It can be recommended for nutrition purposes without fear of harrassment or FDA interference, since they recognize that Spirulina has been eaten for centuries, but they do not allow claims to be made which imply or suggest that it can cure specific diseases.

In Japan and other countries the situation is different and Japanese doctors have even written a book about its use in medical practice, but in the USA this type of research cannot be mentioned in connection with any Spirulina product even if it is true unless it has been tested on animals for several years. So the way to find out is to test it on yourself and write me a letter and tell me what happened, stating whether I can use your letter to inform others of your personal experience. You can also read the Japanese book and make up your own mind and no law can stop you or decide what you can read or what you can do to heal yourself. That is the duty of every person, doctor, scientist or religious minister to "heal thyself".

You might not think that diet and eating has much to do with healing yourself, but it is my personal belief that all diseases, infections and ailments in general start with incomplete nutrition or imbalance. When cells are fed scientifically exact optimum quantities of nutrients they will never die but go on reproducing themselves healthily forever. This is as true for living cells placed in a test tube as it is for a human body. Through my research with algae I have discovered that old age and poor health are the direct result of incorrect diet for the circumstances in the life style. If you are in a situation of stress then your cells are going to be stretched to their limits and beyond, so they need special fortification to withstand it. It is the same with physical stress as with emotional stress. You must build up body, muscles and cells to perform before subjecting them to too much stress. But every weight lifter knows that a certain amount of stress or tension on a muscle is absolutely necessary to bring it up to maximum potential. The same applies to our spiritual lives as to our bodies and cells; unless we stretch our minds and muscles with exercise and feed them with correct nutrients our brains and our circulation systems will not work properly either. Some people live life like hot house plants with all good nutrition but at the first puff of wind they chill or collapse and there is no hardiness. A soft life without challenge is not a healthy life, whatever nutrition is given.

Feeding ourself correctly is a great challenge because everyone is slightly different in their metabolism and everybody's intestine performs a little differently. So there are no experts who can make hard and fast rules about nutrition for everyone. But some things are becoming very clear to leading nutritionists the world over.

The first is that the body must have plenty of protein to get the full range of amino acids which are broken down by our bodies to be recombined in the particular type of proteins which our bodies need. If any one is missing, that specific protein cannot be made or that particular nutrient will not reach its intended site in some hungry cell.

The second is the role of carbohydrates in the biosynthesis of stored energy in the cells. Not all carbohydrates do the same job and many different kinds of sugars are made by the body from the materials we put into it. If we put in sucrose our body has a hard time handling large quantities of it and eventually rebels. If we have glucose and fructose it is not so difficult but the same eventually applies to quantity after awhile. But if we take sugar in the form of glucosides then our liver breaks down what we need and uses the other parts for something else. Certain types of sugar like mannose from kelp and rhamnose from Spirulina are actually helping to metabolize other sugars which have overloaded the bloodstream. In compiling recipes with Spirulina we have taken these factors into account.

My book on fasting with Spirulina called *Rejuvenating the Body Through Fasting With Spirulina Plankton* now has more than 150,000 copies in print and of course is about eating the wonderful Spirulina. But not everyone wants to live permanently on Spirulina, so my student Sonia Beasley has now come up with the answer for gourmet cooks in this recipe book.

I am glad to recommend these dishes now, having tested them, because they are fit for kings. My own diet is more frugal and plain, but I know that when you want to please friends or introduce them to a new source of super nutrition the best thing is to make a gourmet dish of it. Not only that but there are so many culinary artists today that cooking has become a major occupation in our society. There is no doubt about it that humans relate first to their gut, and that applies to gut feelings too!

Hence we are offering Spirulina as a gut-cleansing means to better health and incidentally to many higher things which helped to bring the whole Spirulina saga into human consciousness. It originated in 1967 in an attempt to feed the world by mass photosynthesis but that is another story, and you can read about it if you are inclined to read my other book *Food From Sunlight*.

Food for the mind and spirit of course is more important to some people than food for the gut, but these people are rare. If you should be one of those who have an insatiable appetite for Truth, then this book could be an introduction to a whole range of other types of food for the spirit. (See back of this book.)

But primarily this book is about the best food in the world you can put in your gut and if you eat Spirulina and your body doesn't tell you the same thing within two weeks, I will eat my Spirulina green hat!

Yours nutritionally,

Christopher Hills

WHAT IS SPIRULINA?

Many people call it a "miracle food". They say it has totally changed their life—giving them vibrant health and energy that they never dreamed possible. Although this may be the first time you have heard of Spirulina, it is not new. This incredible substance has been used as a staple for centuries in Chad, in Ethiopia, by the ancient Aztecs, and more recently by the Japanese.

Fresh water algae has the highest conversion rate of sunlight—8%—as compared to other plants (3-5%). Thus it brings you in its most potent form all the nutritional benefits derived from photosynthesis of the sun's light. Spirulina is a small alga that grows naturally in alkaline waters and is cultivated and harvested in hygienic tanks and ponds under the latest scientific conditions. It is a complete vegetable protein and is the source of all the vitamins, minerals, digestive enzymes, trace elements, cell salts and chlorophyll your body needs for perfect nutrition. In fact, it is so power-packed that you could actually live on just two to three teaspoons a day! Spirulina is very concentrated. People's tastes vary, therefore you can adjust the amount of Spirulina in each of these recipes to suit your palette. They still are delicious with half the amount of Spirulina and are excellent even without any. Remember—Spirulina added to any recipe is designed to give you maximum nutrition. By adding one tablespoon of Spirulina to your daily food intake you will be supplied with 20-24 grams of high-quality protein (comparable to 80 grams of meat protein), enough to satisfy the Recommended Daily Allowance (RDA) for a high energy, heavy-duty laborer.

Most of the Spirulina available in this country is harvested from the two-mile wide solar farm at Lake Texcoco, Mexico, at a multi-million dollar facility, Sosa Texcoco, S.A., sponsored by the Mexican government. It is available in tablet form, as pure Spirulina, or combined with other nutritional substances such as ginseng, Brewer's yeast, bee pollen, etc. Pure Spirulina is also available as a powder and can be purchased by the pound, which is the most economical way to use it for cooking. Refer to the back of this book for further information.

BREAKFAST TREATS, SNACKS AND SMOOTHIES

Spirulina smoothies are such a quick way of grabbing a midday snack that's an energy booster as well.

Try the recipes here but also be creative and develop some of your own with your favorite drink combinations. Your children will love the lunchbox snacks such as Sunflower Oomph and Green Yummies and you can feel confident that you're not stuffing them up with empty calories but good, sound nutrition. And the breakfast treats are rich and wonderful—a hearty way to start off the day!

2

SCRAMBLED EGGS WITH TOFU

Gung-ho way to start the day.

6 large eggs
⅓ lb. tofu, mashed
1 cup jack or cheddar cheese, grated
1 tbsp. tamari (soy sauce)
2 tbsp. chopped green onion
1 tbsp. Spirulina
2 medium tomatoes, sliced
1 tbsp. sesame seeds (optional)

1. Beat eggs in a bowl.
2. Add remaining ingredients, except for tomatoes, and mix well.
3. Whisk mixture in skillet over low heat until cheese is melted and eggs reach desired consistency.
4. Serve on platter with tomato slices surrounding the egg mixture.

Serve with whole wheat toast or muffins. The sesame seeds give a delicious nutty crunch.

Serves 4.

SEMOLINA SPIRULINA TREAT

This is a savory type breakfast dish which you will find unusual, but I guarantee very tasty and satisfying, especially on a cold winter morning.

15-20 cashews, chopped coarsely
1 tbsp. vegetable oil
1 tsp. chili seeds (like you have with pizza)
½ tsp. mustard seeds (black, preferably)
2-3 curry leaves*or 1 bay leaf
1 cup semolina (or cream of wheat)
1½ cups buttermilk
salt to taste
1 tbsp. Spirulina

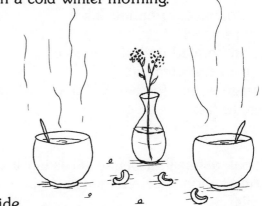

1. Fry the chopped nuts in the oil and then set aside.
2. Fry the red pepper (chili seeds), mustard seeds and curry leaves and stir fry for a minute or so.
3. Turn in the semolina and allow to fry over a moderate flame until golden brown in color.
4. Add the buttermilk, salt and Spirulina.
5. Cook over low flame until all the liquid has been absorbed.
6. Stir in the nuts.
7. Serve warm.

Delicious eaten on its own or with eggs.

Serves 4.

* Curry leaves are available in Indian specialty stores but if they are not to be found in your area, bay leaves will do nicely.

SPIRULINA MUESLI

12 oz. oatmeal or barley flakes
2¼ cups water
juice and grated rind of 1 lemon
4 tbsp. evaporated milk
3 dessert apples (golden Delicious or Pippin)
honey to taste
1½ tbsp. Spirulina

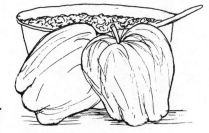

1. Soak oatmeal or barley flakes in water overnight before serving.
2. Add lemon juice and grated rind.
3. Stir.
4. Add milk, stir, grate in well scrubbed apples, including skin and core. Stir frequently to avoid discoloration.
5. Add honey to taste, then put in Spirulina.

This is a basic recipe to which may be added dried fruit, nuts, coconut, etc. This is a most valuable dish, especially for breakfast when the stomach is empty, because its purpose is to stimulate the action of the bacteria in the bowel, making it work more efficiently.

Serves 4.

SUNFLOWER OOMPH

Another de-elicious lunch box goodie.

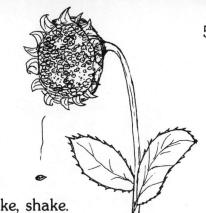

2 cups raw sunflower seeds
2 tsp. Spirulina
½ tsp. vegetable broth mix or to taste
½ tsp. soy sauce
cayenne to taste

Combine the above ingredients together in a plastic bag and shake, shake, shake.

GREEN YUMMIES

Delicious lunch time snack. My son and daughter love them.

2 cups wheatberries, fried or barbecued (available at health food stores)
1 heaped tsp. Spirulina
pinch of cayenne or to taste

1. Put wheatberries in plastic bag.
2. Add rest of ingredients and shake well.

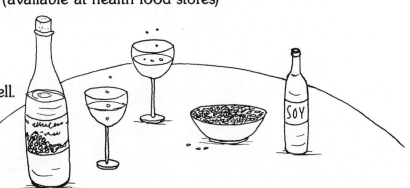

Hey, presto....green yummies.

Serves 4.

SPIRULINA TOASTS

3 sticks (1½ cups) butter
2 crushed garlic cloves
¼ tsp. thyme
2 tbsp. Spirulina
salt and pepper to taste
2 12 in. loaves Italian or French bread
1 cup sesame seeds

1. In a saucepan melt butter with garlic, thyme, Spirulina, salt and pepper.
2. Remove and discard the garlic.
3. Cut bread in ¾ inch slices and dip the slices in the Spirulina/butter mixture.
4. Spread sesame seeds on a sheet of wax paper and roll the bread in the sesame seeds on one side only.
5. Place the slices seeded side up on a baking sheet, bake them in the middle of a preheated oven (400°) for 25-30 minutes or until they are lightly toasted, and arrange them on a bread board.

Serves 6-8.

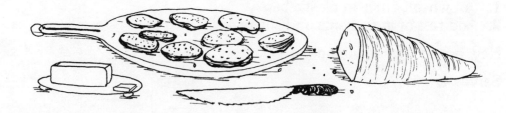

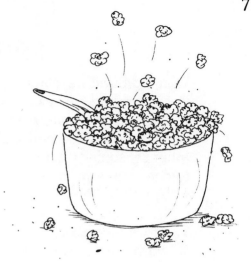

ENERGY POP-POPS

A real favorite in our household.

6 cups popcorn
½ tsp. nutritional yeast
1½ tbsp. Spirulina
your favorite herb
salt to taste
butter

After having popped your corn, add the rest of the ingredients and mix well. Sure is worth the extra time invested.

Serves 6.

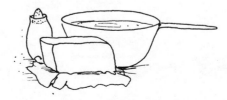

SPIRULINA NUT RISSOLES

½ cup ground hazelnuts
½ cup ground cashew nuts
½ cup whole wheat bread crumbs
½ tsp. fresh mixed herbs, chopped fine (chives, thyme, parsley, etc.)
other seasonings to taste
tomato purée to moisten
1 tbsp. Spirulina

1. Mix all ingredients together to form a stiffish paste.
2. Form into rolls or balls and coat in more ground hazelnuts or almonds.
3. Leave in a cool place for about an hour to absorb all the combined flavors.

Serves 4.

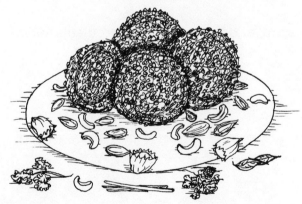

ORANGE COOLERS

Delicious hot weather treat and very eye-appealing.

6 large navel oranges
2 oz. agar agar flakes (available in health food stores)
2 cups water
honey to taste
1 tsp. Spirulina
pinch of salt

1. Cut off tops from oranges and with the aid of a grapefruit knife remove all the orange segments, being careful not to break the skin.
2. Boil together the agar agar and water on low flame till the agar agar is dissolved.
3. Squeeze all the juice out of the removed orange segments and add to the agar agar mixture. Combine with water to make 2½-3 cups liquid.
4. Add honey to taste, salt and Spirulina. Whisk well.
5. Pour liquid into scooped out orange shells and refrigerate for about 1-1½ hours or until set.
6. Quarter the oranges and serve on a bed of lettuce.

Serves 6.

GREEN TARA

1 peach
1 banana
1 pear
1 glass pineapple juice
honey to taste
1 tbsp. Spirulina
2 tbsp. Grapenuts (cereal)

1. Blend all but the last ingredient in blender.
2. Pour into 2 glasses and top with Grapenuts.

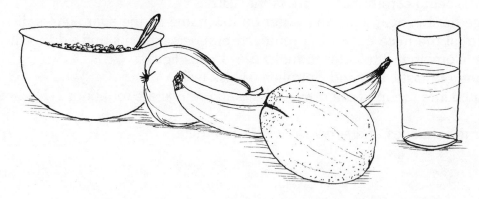

SPIRULINA SMOOTHIE

3 cups apple juice
3 frozen bananas
½ cup frozen blueberries
1½ tbsp. Spirulina
2 tbsp. bran

Blend and drink.
Serves 3.

TROPICAL DELIGHT

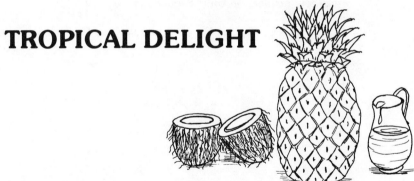

1 cup coconut cream*
3 cups pineapple juice
2 tbsp. cherry syrup
1 tbsp. Brewer's yeast
1 tbsp. Spirulina
2 tbsp. wheat germ

Blend all the above ingredients together in blender and enjoy this tropic delight.
*Coconut cream is not the liquid in coconut. You may grind up the coconut meat and blend with water to make cream. See recipe page 161.
Serves 3.

"Spirulina increased my workouts by 40% and gave me a great burst of energy. I have never experienced this with any other supplement. After having taught two one-hour aerobics classes, I had enough energy to do a two-hour nautilus workout! Spirulina is the best!

M.S.R., Physical Fitness Counselor and Professional Body Builder
Soquel, CA.

DIPS
AND APPETIZERS

Dips and appetizers traditionally are thought of as the naughty little goodies that put on weight. If you go to a cocktail party your downfall is the appetizers, and if you're dieting you try to steer away from them. But the dips and appetizers in this book give you something new in before-dinner eating—food that is actually extra-rich in protein, vitamins and minerals and will contribute to your losing weight instead of gaining it. You'll find these recipes all delicious, and delightful to look at, too!

AVOCADO CREAM DIP

1 large ripe avocado, pitted, peeled
   and cubed
⅓ cup sour cream
1 tbsp. mayonnaise
1 tbsp. lemon juice

1 tsp. grated onion
⅛ tsp. minced garlic
salt and pepper to taste
½ tbsp. Spirulina

1. In a blender or food processor purée the avocado, sour cream, mayonnaise, lemon juice, garlic, onion, salt and pepper and Spirulina.
2. Transfer the cream to a serving bowl.
3. Garnish around the edges of the serving bowl with red pepper, chopped fine.
4. Serve with cold crisp and tender vegetables—cucumber strips, carrots, cauliflower, radishes or any other favorites. Really good.

Makes about 2 cups.

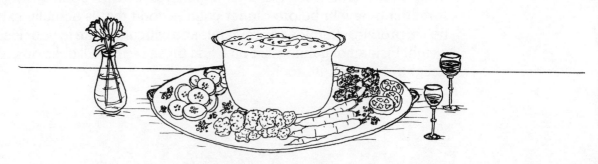

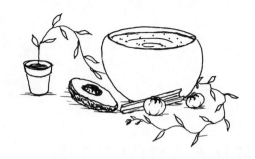

AVOCADO DIPPING SAUCE

1 large avocado
1 lb. sour cream
2 cloves garlic
1 tsp. celery salt (or your favorite)
1 tbsp. Spirulina
any favorite herb or seasoned salt

1. Combine in a blender avocado, sour cream, garlic cloves, celery salt (or your favorite),
   Spirulina and other seasonings.
2. Surround with home grown cherry tomatoes and celery sticks. Delicious chilled.

Makes 2½-3 cups.

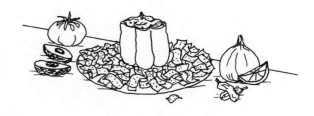

GUACAMOLE DIP

2 tbsp. lemon juice
¾ tsp. salt or to taste
1 small tomato, peeled and cut into small
    pieces
¼ medium onion

2-3 green chili peppers, seeded
2 ripe avocados
1 tbsp. Spirulina
1 large red pepper

1. Blend all ingredients except the pepper in blender till smooth. Stop occasionally and scrape down sides of container with rubber spatula.
2. Special tip: reserve ½ chopped tomato and add to the guacamole after blended.
3. Remove tops and seeds from the red pepper and use it as a bowl for the guacamole.
4. Serve with corn chips—delicious.

Makes about 2½ cups.

DIP A LA SPIRULINA

2 oz. can anchovy fillets, drained
2 tbsp. fresh lemon juice
1 tsp. Dijon style mustard
1 clove garlic
¼ tsp. dried basil

¼ tsp. dried thyme
dash white pepper
¾ cup olive oil
1 tbsp. Spirulina

1. Combine the anchovies, lemon juice, mustard, garlic and seasonings in blender. Cover.
2. Blend on high speed for 30 seconds.
3. Uncover and add oil to mixture in slow steady stream with blender set on high speed.
4. Blend until smooth, about 3 minutes.
5. Spread on toasted French bread slices or serve as a dip with fresh vegetables.

Makes about 1 cup.

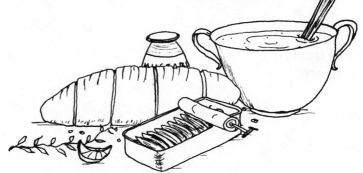

PAM'S GREEN GOOP

1 lb. tofu
Spirulina to taste
miso to taste
spices as desired

    Blend in blender until mayonnaise consistency.

Makes 1 cup.

GREEN GOOP # 2

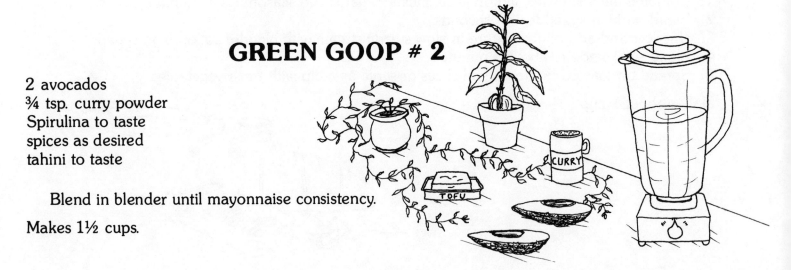

2 avocados
¾ tsp. curry powder
Spirulina to taste
spices as desired
tahini to taste

    Blend in blender until mayonnaise consistency.

Makes 1½ cups.

SPINACH DIPPING SAUCE

Greek, of course!

⅓ lb. feta cheese
1 cup plain yogurt
3 cups minced spinach leaves
¼ cup chopped black olives

3 tbsp. minced green onion
½ tsp. minced garlic
1 tbsp. Spirulina
salt and cayenne to taste

1. Force the feta cheese through a fine sieve into a bowl, whisk in the yogurt and combine the mixture well.
2. Stir in the rest of the ingredients, adding salt to taste.
3. Transfer the sauce to a serving bowl and chill for at least 1 hour.
4. Serve the sauce with toasted pita triangles or raw vegetables.

Makes about 1½ cups.

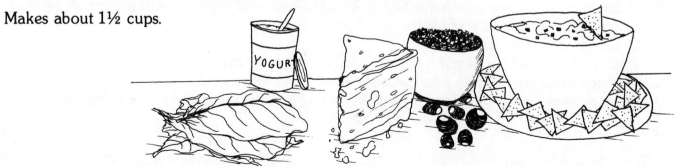

CHEESE BALLS DYNAMITE

Delicious to serve at a cheese and wine party.

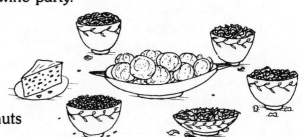

2 medium tomatoes
8 oz. cheddar cheese
3 oz. Weetabix cereal* or wholemeal flakes
1 tbsp. Spirulina
¼ tsp. cayenne or ⅛ tsp. black pepper
¼ lb. almonds, peanuts, pinenuts, pistachios or cashew nuts

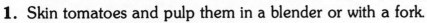

1. Skin tomatoes and pulp them in a blender or with a fork.
2. Crush the Weetabix. Set aside.
3. Grate the cheese, mix together with the Spirulina and bind together with the tomatoes. The mixture should be quite stiff.
4. Divide mixture into equal portions.
5. Flatten each portion and put a nut of your choice in the center.
6. Reshape each portion into a ball and roll in crushed Weetabix.
7. Make at least one hour before serving and stand in a cold place or in the refrigerator.

Makes about 35-40.

*Weetabix is an English whole grain breakfast cereal like Wheaties in this country. Any whole grain flakes will do.

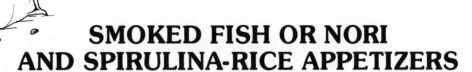

SMOKED FISH OR NORI
AND SPIRULINA-RICE APPETIZERS

1 cup rice (uncooked)
1¼ cups water
2 tsp. soy sauce
2 tbsp. vinegar

1 tsp. honey
½ tsp. salt
1 tbsp. Spirulina
16 thin slices smoked salmon or a packet
   of nori

1. Wash rice and combine with water. Cover and bring to boil.
2. Cook over low heat for 20 minutes or until rice is tender and dry.
3. With a fork stir in the soy sauce, vinegar, honey, Spirulina and salt.
4. Put rice on a board or plate and let it cool completely.
5. Shape teaspoons of the rice mixture into balls or oblong patties.
6. Cut salmon slices in half lengthwise and wrap salmon (or piece of nori) around the rice.

Makes about 32 delectable bites.

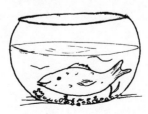

SPIRULINA BITES

A dish similar to falafel.

1½ cups green split peas, soaked overnight
2 oz. onion
2 tsp. cumin seed powder
2 cloves garlic
½ hot pepper or to taste
salt to taste
1½ tsp. Spirulina
oil for deep frying

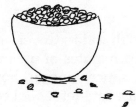
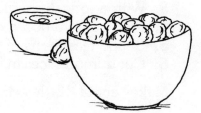

1. Drain soaked peas and reserve one cup of water.
2. Blend the peas in batches in food processor or blender with a little water, some onion, cumin seed, garlic, pepper and salt.
3. Remove each batch as it is processed into a bowl, correct seasonings and add the Spirulina. Stir well.
4. Meanwhile, heat oil until quite hot (not smoking) and fry by dropping teaspoonfuls into the oil, lower oil temperature once the fritter has assumed a firm shape and cook for 2-3 minutes more.
5. Use up all the batter in this way.

These tidbits may be made in advance up to the point of mixing the batter and left unfried or fried and then reheated in a hot oven. Enjoy! Delicious served with mint chutney or any other sweet/hot/sour sauce.

Makes 65-70 bites.

"On the 12th of this month I tried...Spirulina Plankton for the first time. That morning in meditation I had the thought that I needed something for more energy as I had been 'down' for the past six weeks and nothing seemed to do the trick. Later on that day I tried my first teaspoon. I don't think I need tell you what happened....In addition to much greater energy, I've noticed better concentration and even more importantly, a tremendous reduction of stress. So much so that it has been noticeable to many of those around me."

T.H.S., Phoenix, AZ.

SOUPS

Hearty Spirulina soups can be meals in themselves on those busy days when we don't always have time to cook another meal. So fix a big pot and share with your friends, using nice fresh garden vegetables if they're available. Remember not to boil the soup after the Spirulina has been added because it diminishes the potency of the vitamins (although it does not harm the protein content). For added flavor, digestive enzymes and B vitamins add about ¼ cup of miso to any of these recipes. Enjoy!

GREEN GOLD SOUP

A garnish of toasted wheat berries or herbed croutons is a delicious variation.

2 tbsp. oil
½ chopped onion
2 stalks celery, diced or chopped
6 cups vegetable stock
¾ cups split green peas, rinsed
1 bay leaf

6 cups diced zucchini
¼ tsp. basil
⅛ tsp. salt or to taste
1 lb. spinach or watercress, mustard greens
    or any other green
¼ cup fresh chopped parsley
2 tbsp. Spirulina

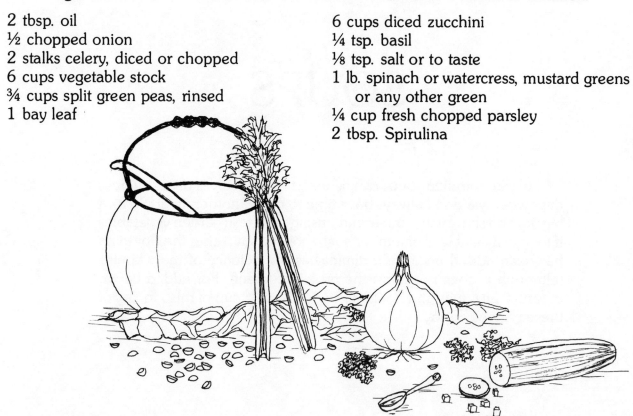

1. Sauté the onion and celery in oil until soft.
2. Add 4 cups of vegetable stock, split peas and bay leaf.
3. Bring to boil, cover and simmer over low heat for about 40 minutes. (Up to this point you could use a pressure cooker.)
4. Add zucchini, remaining 2 cups of stock and seasonings.
5. Cook for another 10 minutes.
6. Remove bay leaf and discard.
7. Purée soup in a blender or food processor.
8. Return to soup pot and add chopped spinach, watercress or other favorite green leaf and parsley.
9. Cook over medium heat for a few minutes.
10. Remove from fire and whisk in Spirulina.
11. Adjust seasonings.

Serves 6-8.

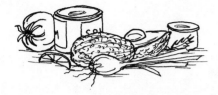

CHILLED SPIRULINA SOUP

Delicious, cool and refreshing.

10½ oz. can condensed consommé
   (chicken or vegetable stock may be used)
2 avocados, peeled and diced
½ cup sour cream (optional)
1 green onion, chopped
1 tsp. salt or to taste

1 tbsp. lemon juice
½ tsp. curry powder
dash hot pepper (optional)
1 tbsp. Spirulina
3 medium tomatoes, peeled and chopped
sour cream
chopped green onion tops or chives

1. Put condensed broth/stock, avocados, sour cream, green onion, salt, lemon juice, curry powder, hot pepper and Spirulina in blender and blend well.
2. Stir in chopped tomatoes and chill thoroughly before serving.
3. To serve, pour into bowls and garnish with a dollop of sour cream and chopped onion tops or chives.

Serves 4-6.

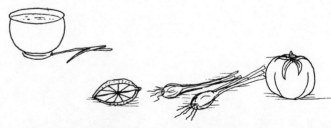

SPIRULINA AZTEC SOUP

This is a delicious and nourishing soup and so easy to prepare.

7 cups boiling water
½ cup tahini
½ cup light yellow miso
¼ cup Spirulina
½ cup picanté sauce or ½ tbsp. cayenne

Combine all ingredients in blender.

Serves 6.

Optional goodies to add after the blending:
    wakame (or hijiki) or arame dried seaweed, soaked in hot water
    onion, garlic
    spinach noodles
    cabbage
    squid, mussels
    diced tofu

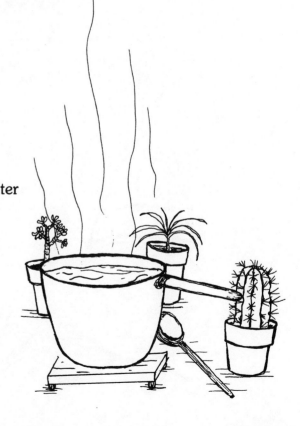

STEPHANIE'S BUSY DAY SOUP

Heat and eat. A speedy treat!

1 qt. V-8 juice
½ cup instant onion
1 tbsp. Spirulina

Combine all ingredients and heat to just below boiling point.

Serves 4.

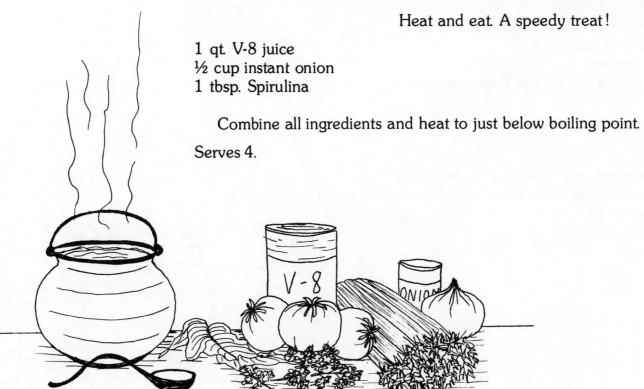

AVOCADO AND WATERCRESS SOUP

Really delicious and full of goodies—iron, vitamins A, B, C, D and Spirulina.

½ tsp. coriander powder
2 ripe avocados
3 cups lightly packed watercress
2 cups chicken or vegetable stock
2 cups heavy cream (light if you prefer)

juice of 1 lemon
1 tbsp. Spirulina
½ tsp. cayenne
½ tsp. salt
½ tsp. pepper
2 tbsp. chopped green onion (strong yellow onion would do)

1. Halve, peel and remove the pits from avocados and cut in pieces.
2. In a blender combine avocado, watercress, stock, Spirulina, cream and green onion and blend the mixture until smooth.
3. Transfer the soup to a bowl and season it with lemon juice, coriander, cayenne, salt and pepper.
4. Chill the soup, covered, for at least 2 hours.
5. Garnish with chopped watercress leaves.

Serves 6-8.

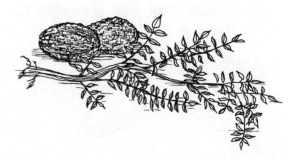

CREAM OF ASPARAGUS SOUP

1 lb. asparagus
4 cups milk, scalded (or you may use vegetable stock)
2 tbsp. butter
2 tbsp. flour
1 tsp. salt
⅛ tsp. pepper
1 tbsp. Spirulina

1. Wash asparagus, cut tips 1½ inches from top. Set aside.
2. Cover remainder of the asparagus with boiling water and cook uncovered until tender.
3. Remove and set aside.
4. Now put in the tips and cook until tender.
5. Remove and set aside.
6. Put in blender the asparagus spears with the liquid and blend till puréed.
7. Set aside.
8. Melt butter in a saucepan, add flour, salt and pepper and pour in asparagus purée.
9. Bring to boil, stirring constantly.
10. Whisk in Spirulina, add asparagus tips and serve hot with whole wheat toast.

Parsley or celery may be used in a similar fashion.

Serves 6.

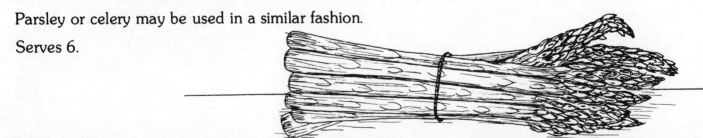

COLD BROCCOLI SOUP

Delicious served with sesame crackers.

1½ lbs. broccoli
4 cups chicken or vegetable stock
¾ cup chopped celery
1 large onion
1 garlic clove
½ tsp. marjoram

1½ tbsp. Spirulina
½ tsp. black pepper
lemon juice to taste
salt to taste
1 tbsp. cornstarch
1 cup light cream (half and half)

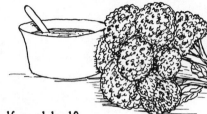

1. Wash the broccoli; cut off the flowerets, reserving a few for garnish.
2. Put the rest in a saucepan with the chicken stock and bring to a boil.
3. Reduce heat and simmer till broccoli is just cooked. Do not over-boil.
4. To this mixture add all the remaining ingredients except the Spirulina and cream.
5. Adjust seasonings and set aside to cool.
6. Add Spirulina and whisk well to avoid lumps from forming.
7. Refrigerate.
8. When ready to serve, pour the cream in gently and stir.
9. Pour into soup bowls and garnish with reserved broccoli flowerets.

This dish is easy to prepare and is light and nutritious because it has a high percentage of vitamins, and with the Spirulina becomes a highly potent protein food.

Serves 6-8.

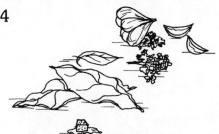

SPIRULINA BASIL SOUP

2 cups firmly packed spinach, sorrel, swiss chard or turnip greens
1 cup firmly packed parsley sprigs
1 cup chicken broth
¾ cup firmly packed basil leaves or ¼ cup dried
¼ cup walnut pieces
1½-2 cloves garlic
¼ cup olive oil
6 cups chicken broth
1 cup orzo (rice shaped pasta) or small noodles
1 egg
½ cup water
2 cups shredded Parmesan cheese
1 tbsp. Spirulina

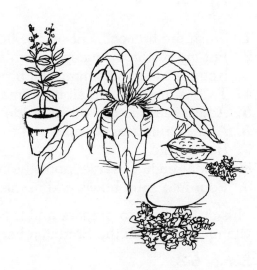

1. Place spinach, parsley, and 1 cup chicken broth in a blender and blend until smooth (2-3 minutes.)
2. Add basil, walnuts, garlic and olive oil and blend until smooth.
3. Pour spinach mixture into saucepan and pour in remaining 6 cups chicken stock.
4. Heat to boiling.
5. Add orzo and return mixture to boil.
6. Reduce heat and simmer, covered, over medium heat until orzo is tender, about 15 minutes.
7. Beat egg with water in medium size bowl, stir in 1 cup of the cheese and Spirulina.
8. Stir 1 cup soup into the egg mixture and then gradually pour the egg mixture into the remaining soup.
9. Serve in individual soup bowls with remaining cheese sprinkled on top.

Serves 6-8.

TOMATO RASAM

This is a drink that we take at the first sign of a cold
or just for the plain enjoyment of a hot/sour drink
which gives you a warm afterglow.

4 cups water

pinch of turmeric

1 tbsp. vegetable oil

¼ cup split peas

12 red onions (or green onions), sliced

4 cloves garlic

1 in. piece cinnamon stick

6 whole black peppercorns

½ lb. ripe tomatoes

juice of ½ lemon

salt to taste

1 tbsp. vegetable oil

6-7 curry leaves* or 2 bay leaves

1½ tbsp. Spirulina

*Curry leaves are available in Indian specialty stores but if they are not
to be found in your area, bay leaves will do nicely.

1. Put water into a pan.
2. When boiling, add turmeric, oil and split peas.
3. Boil together until the split peas are soft.
4. Mash the peas well and strain the liquid.
5. Turn into a pot and add the finely sliced onions, garlic, cinnamon, peppercorns and tomatoes, cut in pieces.
6. Boil.
7. Mash the tomatoes against the sides of the pan and boil again.
8. Strain and add the lemon juice and salt to taste.
9. Put oil into a pan and when hot add the green onions and fry till golden in color.
10. Add the curry leaves and pour the strained Rasam (soup) into it.
11. Remove from fire.
12. Let stand 5-10 minutes.
13. Add Spirulina and whisk well.
14. Serve warm.

Serves 4.

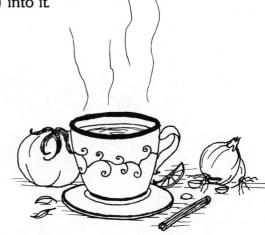

BLACK BEAN SOUP WITH SHRIMP

One of my favorites from Mexico.

3 cups water
¾ cup dried black beans
¼ tsp. oregano
⅛ tsp. ground cumin
1 bay leaf
1 onion, chopped

2 garlic cloves, chopped
2 tbsp. olive oil
1 tomato, peeled and chopped
2 tbsp. Spirulina
2 cups chicken broth or vegetable broth
½ lb. raw shrimp (shelled and cut into ½ inch pieces)
dry sherry

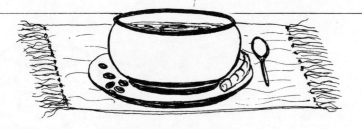

1. Combine the first five ingredients in a saucepan or pressure cooker and cook for about 2 hours (in saucepan) or ½ to ¾ hr. (in pressure cooker). Either way the beans have to be very tender.
2. Remove and discard the bay leaf.
3. Sauté the onion and garlic in olive oil over moderately high heat for 10 minutes, or until onion is soft.
4. Add the peeled and chopped tomato and simmer the mixture, stirring, for 3-4 minutes or until well combined.
5. Season with salt and pepper.
6. Add Spirulina and whisk it in well, so no lumps remain.
7. Add this mixture to the bean mixture.
8. Process in blender to make a pureé.
9. Combine the pureé with the broth in a kettle or Dutch oven and bring the mixture to a simmer over moderate heat.
10. Add the shrimp and simmer the soup for 2-3 minutes.
11. Ladle the soup into heated bowls and stir in 1 tbsp. sherry into each serving.

Delicious served with hot buttered corn tortillas. May be garnished with a sprig of parsley.

Serves 6-8.

SPIRULINA CHIKERINA

6 cups chicken stock
8 oz. packet noodles
4 eggs
meat balls (optional)
½ packet tofu, cut in cubes (optional)
1½ tbsp. Spirulina

1 Bring the stock to a boil.
2. Add noodles and simmer till they are cooked.
3. Beat eggs lightly and stir into soup mixture.
4. Add tofu or cooked meat balls.
5. Whisk in Spirulina and enjoy.

Serves 6.

CHRIS'S SPIRULINA SOUP

3 quarts water
2 tsp. salt
⅓ cup safflower oil
2 onions, thinly sliced, cut in semicircles
6 carrots, diced
2 bunches green onion, diced
¼ cup Spirulina

⅓ cup Brewer's yeast
¼ cup vegetable broth powder
½ cup tahini
3-6 cloves garlic or to taste
¼ cup miso
⅛-¼ tsp. cayenne pepper or to taste
1 handful fresh chopped parsley
4 cups peas, fresh or frozen

1. Bring all but 2 cups of water and salt to boil.
2. Meanwhile, sauté onions, carrots and green onions in oil until onions are transparent.
3. Add to boiling water and simmer until carrots are tender.
4. While this is simmering use a blender to blend with 2 cups water the Spirulina, yeast, vegetable broth powder, tahini, garlic, miso and cayenne. Set aside.
5. Add parsley and peas to onion-carrot brew.
6. Cook for 5 minutes.
7. Add Spirulina blender mix and heat a little longer if necessary. Do not bring the soup to a boil after adding the blender mix.

Suggestion: Crumble rice cakes into bowl. Pour soup over or add cooked grains or cooked noodles.

Serves 10-12.

DELICIOUS SPRING SOUP

6 cups chicken broth
8 oz. fresh sorrel (or spinach)
4 oz. fresh spinach, stems removed
1 bunch watercress, stems removed
¼ cup butter or margarine
¼ cup flour
1 tbsp. Spirulina
1 cup cooked peas
½ cup sour cream
1 tbsp. fresh chives

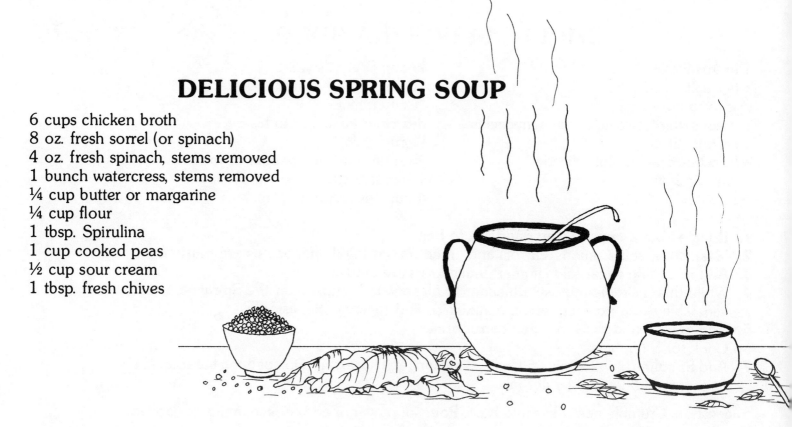

1. Heat chicken broth uncovered in a saucepan over medium heat to boiling.
2. Add sorrel, spinach and watercress and return to boiling.
3. Reduce heat, simmer uncovered for 5 minutes.
4. Cool slightly.
5. Place one-third of the mixture in blender and purée until smooth.
6. Repeat with remaining mixture.
7. Melt butter in saucepan over medium heat.
8. Stir in flour.
9. Cook this mixture, stirring, for 2 minutes.
10. Add puréed mixture gradually.
11. Cook, stirring constantly until thick, about 5 minutes.
12. Whisk in Spirulina and add the hot peas.
13. Simmer, but do not bring to a boil.
14. Combine sour cream and chives.
15. Pour hot soup into individual bowls and top with a spoonful of sour cream mixture.

Serves 8.

GREEN PEA AND WATERCRESS SOUP

A very hearty soup to serve with whole wheat rolls, sitting by a roaring fire.

4 cups green peas (frozen may be used)
5½ cups chicken or vegetable stock
4 cups watercress leaves
1 cup chopped green onion
¼ cup minced mint
1 tsp. chervil
1½ cups cream
2 tbsp. Spirulina
¾ stick butter (3 oz.), softened

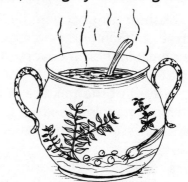

1. Shell peas and put in a saucepan with stock, watercress leaves, chopped green onion, including the green tops, minced mint and chervil.
2. Bring the mixture to a boil and simmer for 30 minutes.
3. Purée the soup in batches in a food processor or blender.
4. Transfer the purée to a saucepan and stir in cream and salt and pepper to taste.
5. Heat soup to just below the boiling point.
6. Whisk in the Spirulina and swirl in the softened butter.
7. Ladle into heated bowls.

Serves 6-8.

SIDE DISHES

In Ceylon many of the curries are treated as side dishes and so we've given you several here as well as other delicious Asian recipes. You'll find the fritters particularly filling and wholesome and you'll send your guests away at the end of the evening with a happy stomach and an extra burst of Spirulina energy!

STUFFED MUSHROOMS

8 large mushrooms
¼ cup butter or margarine
1 tbsp. lemon juice
1 lb. carrots, pared and sliced ¼" thick

¼ tsp. ginger powder
2 tbsp. orange marmalade
1 small onion, finely diced
1 tsp. curry powder
½ tsp. Spirulina

1. Remove stems from mushrooms (reserve for another use) and sauté in butter and lemon juice quickly over moderately high heat until lightly browned, about 3 minutes.
2. Cook carrots in boiling salted water until tender, about 8 minutes. Drain and stir in ginger powder.
3. Purée carrots in electric blender or food processor.
4. Combine orange marmalade, onion, curry powder and Spirulina together and divide evenly among the mushroom caps, filling half full.
5. Squeeze the carrot purée through a pastry bag into the partially filled mushroom caps. (The mushrooms may be refrigerated at this point if made in advance.)
6. Bake in a moderate oven (350°) for 10 minutes or until thoroughly heated.

Serves 8.

FUNCHI

West Indian cornmeal squares.

4 cups water
2 cups yellow cornmeal
2 tsp. salt or to taste
4 tbsp. soft butter
1½ tbsp. Spirulina
minced parsley
radishes, finely sliced

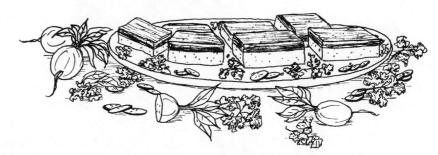

1. In a saucepan bring the water and salt to a boil, sprinkle in the cornmeal, and cook the mixture over moderate heat, stirring until it is thick and leaves the sides of the pan.
2. Divide the cornmeal in half.
3. Beat in 2 tbsp. of the butter into the first half and press the mixture into a buttered 8 inch square baking dish.
4. Mix together the remaining 2 tbsp. of butter with the Spirulina to make a smooth paste.
5. Beat the butter/Spirulina mix into the second half and layer over the first mixture.
6. Let it cool to room temperature and cut into squares.
7. Serve the funchi garnished with minced parsley and finely sliced radishes.

Serves 8.

SALTFISH FRITTERS

Salted cod is available in most supermarkets now, or at specialty stores.

Batter:
⅓ cup flour (whole wheat or white)
⅓ tsp. baking powder
⅓ cup water

Filling:
½ lb. salted cod
4 tbsp. chopped parsley
2 cloves minced garlic
⅛ cup Spirulina
½ tsp. cayenne
salt to taste

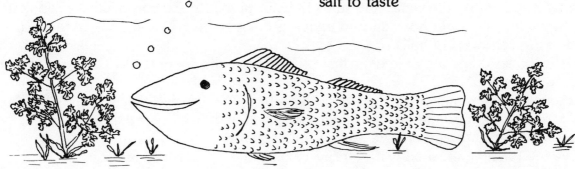

1. Soak cod overnight and flake or shred it.
2. To the above basic batter add one cup cod, well-packed, parsley, garlic, Spirulina, cayenne and salt.
3. Mix well and drop by teaspoons into hot deep fat. Fry till mixture rises to surface.
4. Drain well and serve hot.

Makes about 40-50 fritters (serves 10-15).

You may also use other ingredients such as ¾ to 1 cup chopped ham; 1 small onion, grated; 1 green pepper, seeded and finely chopped and ⅛ cup Spirulina. Follow the above procedure.

OR 1 cup cooked minced chicken or turkey, 1 tsp. black pepper, 3 tbsp. chopped parsley, 3 tbsp. chopped celery, 1 small onion, grated and ⅛ cup Spirulina. Even hardboiled eggs may be incorporated into this batter.

These bites are quite delicious and I find they are the first to disappear at any of the parties where I have served them.

CAULIFLOWER STUFFED TOMATOES

6 large tomatoes, ripe and firm
1 large cauliflower (approx. 3 lbs.)
3 tbsp. tarragon vinegar
3 tbsp. dry white wine
3 tbsp. minced shallots
1 tbsp. heavy cream

3 large egg yolks, lightly beaten
1 cup clarified butter (see recipe p. 67)
lemon juice
salt and pepper to taste
1 tsp. Spirulina
parsley sprigs
radishes

1. Halve the tomatoes decoratively, and with a teaspoon or a demitasse spoon, seed, core and juice them, without squeezing them.
2. Sprinkle the tomatoes with salt and let them drain, inverted, on paper towels for 30 minutes.
3. Trim and separate the cauliflower into flowerets and cook for 4-6 minutes in a large saucepan of boiling salted water.
4. Drain, cover, and keep warm.
5. In a small stainless steel pan combine the vinegar, wine and minced shallots.
6. Simmer on high heat until liquid is reduced to 1 tablespoon. Remove from heat.
7. Add cream and egg yolks to the tablespoon of liquid and cook the mixture over low heat, stirring constantly, until thick.
8. Whisk in clarified butter, 2 tablespoons at a time, removing the pan occasionally from the heat to cool the mixture.
9. Stir until thick.
10. Strain the sauce through a fine sieve into another bowl and add the lemon juice, salt and pepper.
11. Add Spirulina and whisk in well till smooth and shiny. Keep warm, covered, in a shallow pan of hot water.
12. Arrange the tomatoes on a plate and divide the cauliflower flowerets among them.
13. Carefully spoon sauce over the cauliflower and sprinkle with finely chopped radishes and surround with parsley.

Serves 12.

PINEAPPLE CURRY

An excellent accompaniment to rice and chicken curry and salad.

2-2½ lb. pineapple
1 tbsp. peeled, chopped fresh ginger
5 garlic cloves
¾ cup chopped onion
1 sliced green pepper (hot or mild, as
    desired)
salt to taste
1½ tsp. pepper
¼ tsp. turmeric

2 tbsp. vegetable oil
½ cup thinly sliced onion
2" piece cinnamon stick
¼ crushed cardamon seed
3-4 curry leaves or 1 bay leaf
½ cup honey
¼ cup raisins
2 tbsp. flour
1 cup coconut milk (or regular milk)
1 tbsp. rosewater (available in drug store)
1 tbsp. Spirulina

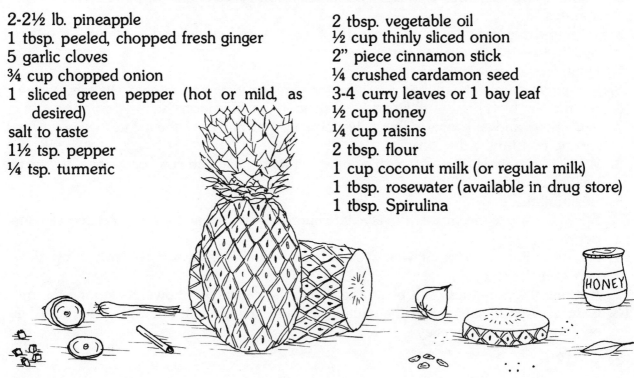

1. Twist the leaves from an underripe pineapple, peel and core the pineapple and cut into cubes.
2. In a blender or food processor grind the ginger, garlic, chopped onion, sliced pepper, salt, pepper and turmeric.
3. Heat the oil in a saucepan over moderately high heat until it is hot, add sliced onion, cinnamon, cardamon and curry leaves and sauté the mixture until onion is golden.
4. Stir in pineapple and ginger/garlic mixture, reduce heat to low and cook for 20 minutes, or until the liquid has evaporated.
5. Stir in the honey and raisins and cook, stirring constantly, until honey is absorbed.
6. In a small bowl mix the flour with the coconut milk and pour onto the pineapple mixture.
7. Simmer the mixture, stirring occasionally, for 15 minutes.
8. Remove pan from heat and stir in the rosewater and Spirulina.

Serves 4-6.

A word about coconut milk. We in Ceylon use it because of the unique flavor it imparts to all the food that it is cooked in. So if you do substitute regular milk for it, the flavor will not be the same.

WALNUT SPIRULINA RICE

Super good!

1 cup brown rice
2 large onions, chopped
2 tbsp. tomato purée
1 tbsp. sage
1 tbsp. parsley
1 tbsp. chopped celery

salt and pepper to taste
4 oz. ground walnuts
1 egg
1¼ tbsp. Spirulina
sliced almonds
coconut flakes

1. Cook rice in 2 cups water in usual manner.
2. While rice cooks (until tender but NOT mushy) fry onions until soft.
3. Add tomato purée and fry a little.
4. Add sage, parsley, celery, salt and pepper.
5. Add cooked rice to onion/tomato mixture.
6. Add Spirulina and all other ingredients.
7. Cover and keep warm.
8. Garnish with sliced almonds and coconut flakes.

Serves 4.

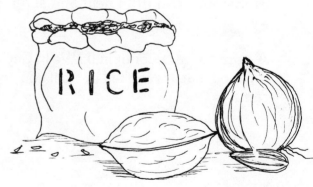

AVOCADO MOUSSE

Delicious served with thinly sliced buttered whole wheat bread.

2 ripe avocados
½ cup olive oil
¼ cup lemon juice
salt and pepper to taste
1 tbsp. Spirulina
3 tbsp. heavy cream
3 tbsp. mayonnaise

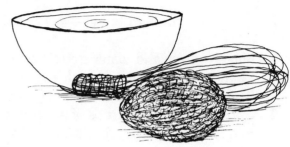

1. Peel, halve and cut the avocados into thin slices.
2. Combine the olive oil, lemon juice, salt and pepper to taste and add in the avocado slices. Let them marinate for about 1 hour.
3. Transfer the avocados and marinade to a blender and purée the mixture.
4. Combine the mixture with the cream, mayonnaise and Spirulina and beat with a wire balloon whisk until light and fluffy.
5. Add more lemon juice to taste.
6. Divide the mousse among 6 individual dishes and lay overlapping thin slices of cucumber around each portion.

I've found this to be a quick and easy dish to whip up when I have a friend over without much advance notice. It will always forestall the hunger pangs and it gives you a quick energy boost.

Serves 6.

STUFFED PARATHAS

Dough:

2 cups whole wheat flour
1 cup water
½ tsp. salt
1 tbsp. ghee (clarified butter—see recipe p. 67)

1. Make a flour and water dough with the above ingredients.
2. Put flour into a bowl, add salt and gradually add water, mixing until a soft dough is formed.
3. Knead well with the fist, folding and kneading until dough is pliable.
4. Sprinkle with a few drops of water, cover with a damp tea towel and leave to stand for a few minutes (if in a hurry), otherwise for a minimum of 30 minutes.

Stuffing:

2-3 lbs. potatoes
2 tbsp. ghee or oil
1 onion, finely chopped
2 tbsp. fresh coriander leaf (Spanish parsley) or parsley
½ in. piece ginger, finely chopped
1 clove garlic, finely chopped
salt to taste
½ tsp. garam masala (available at any Indian food store)
¼ tsp. chili powder
1 tsp. lemon juice
1 head of any type of green leaf (spinach, lettuce) finely shredded
2 tsp. Spirulina

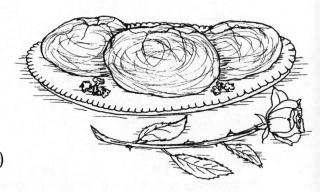

1. Boil potatoes and when cool, peel and mash.
2. Heat ghee or oil and fry the onion, herbs and ginger and garlic for a few minutes.
3. Add salt, garam masala and chili powder.
4. Mix the mashed potato, shredded lettuce, Spirulina and lemon juice.
5. Mix all ingredients together well. Remove from heat and allow to cool slightly.
6. Meanwhile, divide the paratha dough into 6 balls.
7. Roll each dough ball into a flat round the size of a saucer and place 1-2 tbsp. of the potato mixture in the center.
8. Bring the sides of the paratha up until you have a round ball in your hand.
9. Leave to set, and continue following this procedure until you have used up all the dough and the potato mixture.
10. Flour a pastry board and place the filled dough on it.
11. Roll gently to about a 6-8 inch round.
12. Heat an iron griddle on medium heat to warm up.
13. Grease slightly and place the stuffed parathas on it.
14. Sprinkle a dab of ghee on the side of paratha facing you and keep turning occasionally so as not to burn the paratha. It usually puffs up when ready. Care must be taken when rolling not to break the skin of the paratha, otherwise it will burst open and will not puff up.

Paratha is a very basic Indian unleavened bread. This recipe is only one way to make it; you could also use peas, mashed cauliflower, carrots, etc. in the stuffing if you so wish.

Makes 6-8.

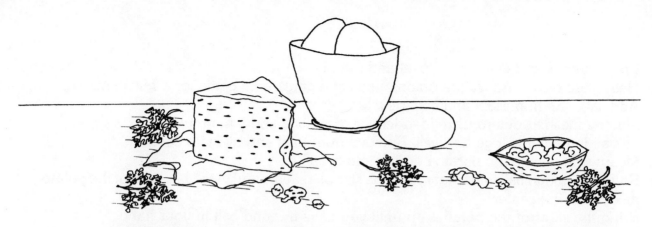

CELERY, WALNUT, SPIRULINA FRITTERS

¾ lb. Stilton cheese or any bleu cheese of
   your choice
¾ cup minced celery
¾ cup minced walnuts
¾ cup minced water chestnuts

6 tbsp. fresh chopped parsley
¼-½ tsp. cayenne (optional)
1 tbsp. Spirulina
3 eggs
oil for deep frying
1-2 cups bread crumbs

1. Combine the first 7 ingredients and mix well.
2. Keep covered in refrigerator until firm.
3. Divide mixture into equal portions and form in balls the size of a walnut.
4. Beat eggs lightly and roll the balls in egg wash and then in bread crumbs. If they have become too soft in the rolling process, put on plate and chill again until firm.
5. Fry the fritters in batches in deep hot oil for about 3 minutes or until golden.

Makes about 24 melt-in-the-mouth delights.

SPIRULINA ZUCCHINI FRITTERS

Serve with a fresh green salad with your favorite homemade tomato or sweet/hot sauce.

1 lb. zucchini, shredded large
3 eggs
3 tbsp. cornmeal
3 tbsp. whole wheat flour
¼ cup Spirulina
¾ cup chopped parsley
½ head romaine lettuce, shredded
1 tsp. black pepper
½ tsp. whole cumin seed
½ tsp. celery salt or to taste
2 cloves crushed garlic

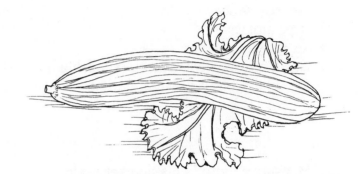

1. Combine all the above ingredients and mix well together.
2. Taste for seasoning and adjust.
3. Heat a skillet with about 3 inches vegetable fat and drop the fritter mixture in by tablespoons.
4. Cook for about 2-3 minutes and turn over.
5. Following the same procedure, continue frying till all the batter is used up.

These are very tasty as a side dish, or if you prefer to make it a more wholesome meal just add ½ cup of peanuts or sunflower seeds to the batter and follow the same procedure.

Makes about 15-20 fritters (serves 6-8).

FISH ROLLS

Sauce:
3 tbsp. melted butter
2 tbsp. soy sauce
1½ tsp. molasses
½ tsp. ginger powder
½ tsp. Chinese Five Spices (available in Oriental section of supermarket)

Fish mixture:
6 fillets of plaice (sole)
½ lb. crab meat
3 finely chopped green onions
1 tsp. chopped parsley
1 tbsp. Spirulina
1 tbsp. butter
1 clove crushed garlic
salt and pepper to taste
½ tsp. lemon juice

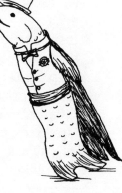

1. Mix sauce ingredients and set aside.
2. Place fillets of plaice between 2 sheets of wax paper and flatten. Set aside.
3. Mix together the crab meat, green onions, parsley, Spirulina, garlic, butter, salt, pepper and lemon juice.
4. Divide this mixture into 6 parts and form an elongated roll and place on a fish fillet.
5. Roll fillet and secure with a toothpick.
6. Place rolls in a compact oven-proof dish and pour the sauce over the fish.
7. Bake in a moderate oven (350°) for ½ hour to 45 minutes.
8. Slice each fillet into 6 or 7 slices and serve on a bed of buttered brown rice.

Makes about 40.

SPINACH BALLS

1½ lbs. spinach
½ tsp. fresh ginger, finely chopped
1 green chili (optional)
4 cloves garlic
½ tsp. salt
1 tbsp. Spirulina
½ tsp. curry powder
flour

1. Wash spinach and cook for a few minutes with water that clings to leaves from washing.
2. Strain well and purée in liquidizer.
3. Add rest of ingredients and enough flour to make a stiff mixture.
4. Roll into balls and deep fry.
5. Serve hot with your favorite curry sauce.

Serves 4.

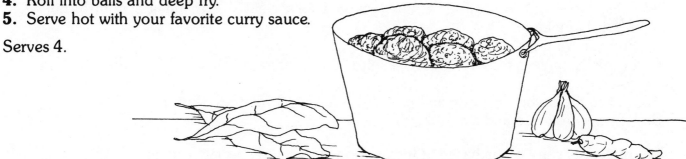

CASHEW CURRY

1 lb. unsalted raw cashews, whole
1 tsp. baking soda
2 cups coconut milk (or half coconut milk
 and half regular milk.) Recipe follows.
2-3 curry leaves*or 1 bay leaf
1 tbsp. minced fresh ginger

¼ tsp. cayenne
salt to taste
6 shallots
3 tbsp. oil
1 tbsp. Spirulina

1. Soak cashews in cold water to cover with the baking soda for about 1-1½ hours.
2. Drain.
3. In a saucepan combine nuts with the milk, curry leaves, ginger, cayenne and salt.
4. Bring the mixture to a boil and simmer, covered, for about 15-20 minutes, or until the nuts are just tender.
5. Remove from fire.
6. In a skillet sauté in the oil 6 shallots, thinly sliced, over moderately high heat until they are golden.
7. Add to the cashew mixture and cook for a further 3 minutes, stirring.
8. Remove from fire and stir in the Spirulina.

*Curry leaves can be purchased at Indian food stores and specialty shops.

Coconut Milk:

1. In a saucepan combine 4 cups water and 3 cups grated fresh coconut.
2. Bring the water to a boil, stirring, remove pan from heat, and let the mixture sit for about 30-45 minutes.
3. Strain through a sieve lined wth dampened cheesecloth, squeezing the cheesecloth to extract all the liquid.

   OR

1. Put 3 cups water and 2 cups fresh grated coconut into the blender.
2. Cover and process at medium speed for 2 minutes.
3. Strain through cheesecloth, making sure to extract all the liquid.

Makes about 3 cups.

The Cashew Curry should be served with rice and meat or fish curry, chutney and salad.

Serves 4.

64

VITAMIN B12 AND SPIRULINA

You can receive the RDA of Vitamin B12 from only 5 tablets of Spirulina (500 mg.). In fact, 4 tablets of Spirulina give the same amount of Vitamin B12 as two 8-ounce glasses of milk, or two eggs, or a cup of cottage cheese. Gram for gram, Spirulina has 2½ times more Vitamin B12 than liver.

VITAMIN A AND SPIRULINA

Four ounces of liver provide 50,000 International Units of Vitamin A. Spirulina provides 26% more Vitamin A in one heaped tablespoon (63,000 I.U.). One teaspoonful of Spirulina contains twice the Vitamin A of a carrot.

IRON AND SPIRULINA

One heaped tablespoon (20 grams) of Spirulina has 11.6 mg. of iron, more than 3 times the iron in a 4 ounce sirloin steak (3.7 mg.).

MAIN DISHES— VEGETARIAN

The concern for most vegetarians is to find a good source of protein for their diet, and until now they have often turned to soybeans as their solution. But many have now switched to Spirulina because of all of its added life-giving and energy-building properties.

Wondrous things can be done with the simple little garden vegetable to make it into a substantial main attraction of any meal. And with the addition of Spirulina you and your guests leave the table feeling filled and happy inside because your body knows that its nutritional needs have been met. Turn the humble pea into an elegant Summer Peas Pudding or try an exotic, spicy Curd Curry....all of these dishes have received enthusiastic hoorays from the many who have tried them.

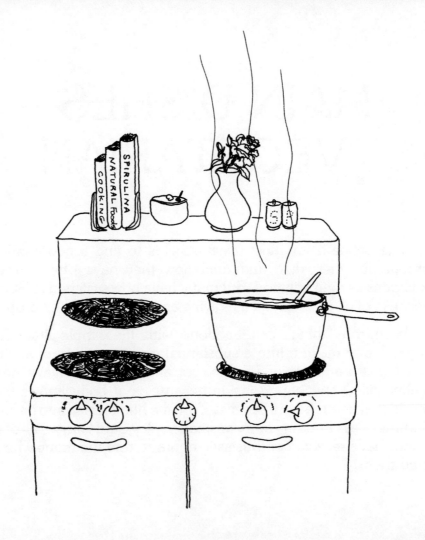

Several of the recipes in this book call for clarified butter. This is how you make it.

CLARIFIED BUTTER (or Ghee)

1. In a heavy saucepan over low heat melt 2 sticks (1 cup) unsalted butter which has been cut into 1 inch pieces.
2. Remove pan from the heat and let the butter stand for about 3 minutes.
3. Skim the froth from the surface and strain the butter through a sieve, lined with a double thickness of rinsed and squeezed cheesecloth, into a bowl, leaving the milky solids in the bottom of the pan.
4. Pour the clarified butter into a jar or a crock and cover. Clarified butter will keep indefinitely when covered and chilled. It loses about one-fourth of its original volume.

Yield: ¾ cup clarified butter.

SPINACH LOAF WITH MUSHROOM SAUCE

2 lbs. fresh spinach or chard (stems removed)
½ cup chopped green onion with tops
3 tbsp. butter or margarine
4 eggs
1 cup half and half

1 tsp. salt or to taste
½ tsp nutmeg
½ tsp. pepper
⅔ cup dry whole wheat bread crumbs
½ cup grated Parmesan cheese
3 tbsp. sesame seeds

1. Place spinach in Dutch oven, retaining the water that clings to leaves from washing.
2. Steam, covered, over medium heat until spinach is limp, about 4 minutes.
3. Drain.
4. Rinse in cold water, pressing out excess moisture in strainer.
5. Chop and put aside.
6. Sauté green onion in butter in small skillet until transparent, about 3 minutes.
7. Combine eggs, half and half and seasonings in a large bowl.
8. Stir in spinach, onion, bread crumbs, cheese and sesame seeds.
9. Spoon spinach mixture into a well greased loaf pan (9 x 5 x 3) or ring mold.
10. Place pan in a shallow baking pan.
11. Pour 2 inches of hot water into the larger pan.
12. Bake in a preheated 350° oven until knife inserted in center comes out clean, 1-1¼ hours.
13. Remove pan from water and let stand 5-10 minutes.
14. Unmold spinach loaf onto serving platter. Serve with Mushroom Spirulina Sauce.

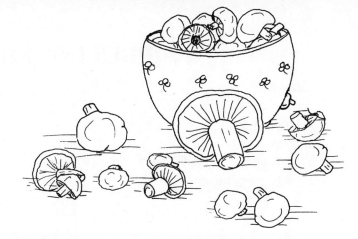

Mushroom Spirulina Sauce:

1 cup fresh mushrooms, thinly sliced
6 tbsp. butter or margarine
3 tbsp. flour
½ tsp. salt or to taste
½ tsp. pepper
1 cup half and half
1 tbsp. Spirulina

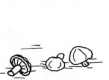

1. Sauté mushrooms in 3 tbsp. of the butter in a small skillet over medium heat for 3 minutes or until tender.
2. Melt remaining butter in a 1 quart saucepan over medium heat.
3. Stir in flour, salt and pepper.
4. Cook and stir 2 minutes.
5. Add half and half gradually, whisking so no lumps remain, until mixture thickens, about 5 minutes.
6. Stir in Spirulina and blend well.
7. Stir in mushrooms.

Serves 8.

SPIRULINA FILLED CRÊPES

Crêpes:
1 cup water
½ cup milk
2 eggs
1 cup whole wheat flour
2 tbsp. vegetable oil
salt to taste

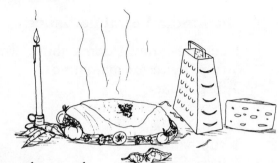

1. Blend water, milk, eggs, flour, oil and salt in blender until smooth.
2. Refrigerate, covered, for about 2 hours for best results.
3. Heat lightly greased crêpe pan or skillet over medium heat.
4. Pour about 3 tbsp. of batter into pan.
5. Tilt pan quickly and coat bottom evenly with batter.
6. Cook until lightly browned, about 2 minutes on each side.
7. Stack crêpes till all the batter has been used up.

Filling:
10 oz. fresh or frozen spinach
2 tbsp. butter or margarine
2 tbsp. whole wheat flour
½ tsp. salt
½ tsp. nutmeg
½ tsp. freshly ground pepper

½ cup whipping cream
1 tbsp. Spirulina
½ cup shredded Swiss cheese
grated Parmesan cheese (optional)
parsley sprigs and cherry tomatoes (optional)

1. Place spinach in Dutch oven with water that clings to the leaves from washing.
2. Steam, covered, over medium heat until just limp, about 2 minutes.
3. Drain.
4. Rinse in cold water.
5. Press out any excess moisture in strainer.
6. Chop.
7. Melt butter in 2 quart saucepan over medium heat.
8. Stir in flour, salt, nutmeg, pepper.
9. Cook and stir over medium heat about 2 minutes.
10. Add cream gradually.
11. Cook, stirring constantly, until mixture thickens, about 2 minutes.
12. Stir in the chopped spinach, Spirulina and Swiss cheese.
13. Heat oven to 350°.
14. Spoon about 1 tbsp. of spinach mixture onto center of each crêpe; roll up.
15. Arrange in single layer in baking dish.
16. Bake until warm, about 10 minutes.
17. Sprinkle with Parmesan cheese and garnish with parsley sprigs and cherry tomatoes.

Makes 12-14.

EGGS FLORENTINE À LA SPIRULINA

1½ lbs. spinach
½ tsp. celery salt
½ tsp. Lawry's Salt
2 oz. butter
1 tbsp. Spirulina
¼ cup flour
¾ pt. milk

3 oz. grated Parmesan or cheddar cheese
6 eggs
3 tbsp. light cream
tomato slices

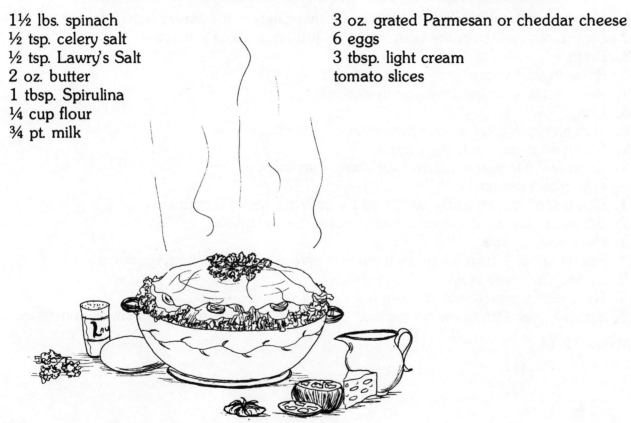

1. Wash spinach and chop roughly.
2. Put into bowl with a little salt and just the water that clings to the leaves.
3. Mix with 1 oz. of the butter, seasonings and Spirulina.
4. Put into an oven-proof dish.
5. Make a cheese sauce: melt the remaining butter in a pan, blend in the flour and cook over a gentle heat for 1 minute.
6. Remove pan from heat, stir in milk and bring to boil, stirring.
7. Cook for a further 2 minutes.
8. Stir in 2 oz. of the cheese. Do not cook again.
9. Poach the eggs lightly and place side by side on spinach.
10. Add cream to the cheese sauce and pour over the spinach and eggs.
11. Sprinkle with remaining cheese.
12. Put dish in the center of a moderate oven (375°) and bake 10 to 15 minutes or until golden brown. (An alternative is to brown under the broiler.)
13. Garnish with tomato slices.

You may boil the eggs soft or hard to vary this dish. You may also use frozen spinach if you wish.

Serves 6.

EMERALD ISLE AVOCADO

1 green pepper, diced
1 tbsp. butter or oil
6-8 mushrooms, sliced
1 cup heavy cream
3 avocados
1 egg yolk, lightly beaten
2 tbsp. Spirulina
salt and pepper to taste
lemon juice

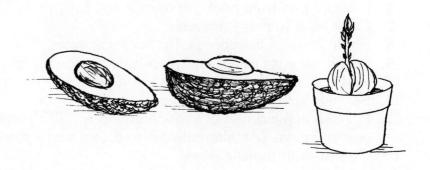

1. Sauté green pepper in oil over moderate heat for 3-4 minutes, or until soft.
2. Add sliced mushrooms and cook for a further minute.
3. Pour off oil.
4. Add cream and bring to boil.
5. Halve avocados lengthwise and remove pits.
6. Scoop out flesh in large pieces, taking care not to tear the shells. Reserve shells.
7. Cut flesh into cubes.
8. Add avocado to vegetable mixture and cook over moderate heat for 8-10 minutes or until the sauce is thickened.
9. Remove pan from heat and stir in the egg yolk, Spirulina, salt and pepper to taste.
10. Add lemon juice if desired.
11. Fill shells with mixture and put them under a preheated broiler for 30-45 seconds or until the tops are glazed.

For a richer dish add shrimp, lobster, cubed ham or chicken.

Serves 6.

GREEN PEPPER/TOMATO SAUTÉ

And of course, an ice cold beer!

1½ large onions, chopped
⅓ cup olive or vegetable oil
3 large green peppers, cut lengthwise into ¼" strips
3 large cloves crushed garlic
1½ tsp. salt or to taste
½-1 tsp. honey
½ tsp. pepper
5 medium tomatoes, cut in wedges
1½ tbsp. Spirulina

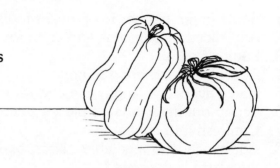

1. Sauté onions in oil in large skillet over medium heat until tender, about 3 minutes.
2. Stir in pepper strips.
3. Sauté, stirring occasionally until peppers are crisp/tender, about 10 minutes.
4. Stir in remaining ingredients except tomato wedges, mixing well.
5. Place tomato wedges on top of pepper mixture and cook gently for 2 minutes.
6. Stir in tomatoes.
7. Serve on bed of brown rice and salad.

Serves 6-8.

BE BE'S PIZZA

2 cups whole wheat flour
½ cup oil
¼ cup water
1-2 tsp. Spirulina
½ cup olives
½ cup mushrooms

1 cup mozzarella cheese, grated
1 medium onion, chopped
1 large green pepper, chopped
1 cup grated zucchini (optional)
¼ lb. tofu, cubed (optional)
Italian seasoning to taste
15½ oz. can marinara sauce

1. Mix flour, oil, water and Spirulina and form into ball.
2. Roll out between 2 pieces of waxed paper to about ⅛" thickness.
3. Place on ungreased cookie sheet and pile on vegetables.
4. Sprinkle on spices, marinara sauce and grated cheese.
5. Bake in preheated 350° oven for 10-15 minutes or until done.

Makes one medium pizza.

OLÉ PILAF

Pretty to look at. Yummy to eat!

2 cups buckwheat groats (kasha) or bulgar
2 cups chopped tomato
1 cup cooked peas (fresh or frozen)
1 tbsp. chili powder
1 tsp. salt or to taste
pepper to taste
1 cup chopped celery
½ lb. mushrooms, quartered
1 cup chopped onion
½ stick butter, or oil and butter combination
½ tsp. oregano
1½ tbsp. Spirulina
½ lb. grated sharp cheddar cheese
1 red pepper, cut in strips

1. Cook groats in vegetable or chicken stock.
2. Combine the groats in a bowl with the chopped tomato, peas, chili powder, salt and pepper.
3. In a skillet sauté the celery, mushrooms and onion in the butter over moderately high heat for about 4-5 minutes, or until they are tender.
4. Combine the vegetables with the buckwheat or bulgar mixture, add oregano and test for seasonings.
5. Transfer mixture to a buttered gratin dish, cover, and bake in a preheated 350° oven for 30 minutes.
6. Remove from oven and sprinkle in Spirulina and top with the grated cheese.
7. Put the dish under a preheated broiler until cheese melts and is golden brown.
8. Garnish with strips of red pepper in a flower design.

Serves 6.

VEGETABLE STUFFED TOMATOES

Good served with fresh green salad, pita bread and mint/yogurt chutney
(mix 1 pint yogurt with ½ cup mint sauce).

Stuffing:

6 medium tomatoes
1 tsp. brown sugar
3 oz. cooked green peas (fresh or frozen)
3 oz. cooked diced carrots
3 oz. cubed tofu (fried) or potatoes
salt to taste
1 oz. cooking oil
1 oz. finely chopped green onion

½ tsp. chopped ginger
1 green pepper, chopped
¼ tsp. red pepper or cayenne
1 tbsp. chopped coriander leaves (Spanish parsley)
1 tbsp. chopped parsley
1 tbsp. chopped mint
1½ tbsp. Spirulina

Batter:

¼ cup whole wheat flour
5 tbsp. water
pinch of salt
pinch of black pepper
oil for frying

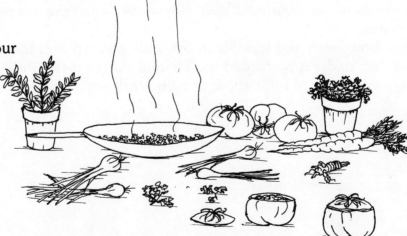

1. Cut off a slice from the top of each tomato and set aside.
2. Scoop out pulp and drain off tomatoes by laying them upside down on paper towels.
3. Heat the oil and fry onions lightly.
4. Add tomato pulp and cook until dry.
5. Add sugar, cooked peas, carrots, potatoes or tofu, salt, green onion and seasonings.
6. Cook until spices penetrate the vegetables.
7. Remove from fire and add Spirulina.
8. Pile this mixture into the tomato shells and replace cut slices back as lids.
9. Mix all batter ingredients together, dip tomatoes in carefully, and deep fry for a minute or so.
10. Serve immediately.

These may instead be baked after stuffing for ease of preparation, in which case add Spirulina to the stuffing mix.

Serves 6.

SPIRULINA STUFFED EGGPLANT

6 eggplants, about 3" long
6 bunches green onions
2 tbsp. oil plus 2 tbsp. butter or margarine
3 cloves minced garlic
1 medium onion, chopped
1½ cups cooked brown rice
1 cup shrimp, minced clams or ground beef
    (optional)
¼ cup Spirulina

¼ cup minced parsley
1 tsp. chopped basil
¼ tsp. chopped thyme
2 tbsp. Worcestershire sauce
3 tbsp. tomato ketchup
1 tsp. Tabasco or to taste
1 cup Gruyère or cheddar cheese
salt and black pepper to taste

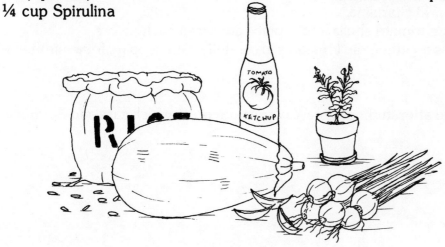

1. Halve the eggplants lengthwise and scoop out the pulp, leaving a ¼" shell.
2. Sprinkle the shells with salt and invert them on paper towels to drain.
3. Chop the pulp.
4. In a skillet sauté the green onions, including the tops, in oil/butter.
5. Add minced garlic, onion and the chopped eggplant and continue cooking for about 10 minutes or until the eggplant is softened.
6. Add the cooked rice, shrimp, clams or beef, Spirulina, parsley, basil, thyme, sauces and salt and pepper.
7. Stir and mix well.
8. Adjust seasonings.
9. Fill eggplant shells with the stuffing.
10. Arrange stuffed eggplants on a buttered baking dish.
11. Top with cheese and bake in a preheated moderately hot oven (370°) for 25-30 minutes or until cheese is golden.
12. Serve with a fresh tossed salad.

Serves 6 as a main dish or 12 as a first course.

HERBED TOMATOES

6 firm ripe medium tomatoes
salt and pepper to taste
2 tbsp. oil
⅔ cup flat leaf parsley, minced
⅔ cup fresh bread crumbs
⅔ cup freshly grated Parmesan cheese
2 tbsp. Spirulina
2 cloves minced garlic
1 tsp. celery salt

1. Cut tomatoes in half and gently scoop out the seeds and the liquid without squeezing the tomatoes.
2. Sprinkle with salt and pepper and brush with oil.
3. Arrange the tomatoes cut side up on a lightly oiled baking sheet and bake them in a preheated oven (325°) for 20 minutes.
4. Invert the tomatoes onto a rack and let them drain for at least 30 minutes.
5. Combine the rest of the ingredients in a bowl.
6. Divide the mixture equally among the tomatoes, mounding it.
7. Drizzle with oil, arrange on the rack of a broiler pan, and broil them under a preheated broiler about 5 inches from the heat for 5 minutes, or until the filling is bubbly and lightly golden.
8. Sprinkle with more salt and pepper if desired.

Serves 6.

HARVEY'S VEGETABLE HIGHLIGHT

2 large zucchinis or 12 small ones
2 large onions
8 carrots
2 cabbages
1 cup sesame oil
6 tbsp. tamari
5 tsp. Spirulina

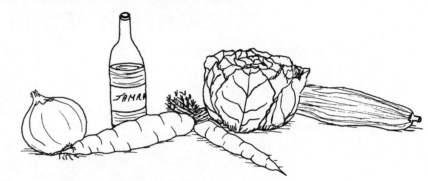

1. Chop zucchini, onions and carrots.
2. Heat oil to hot temperature in frying pan and add these ingredients.
3. Stir well and fry 2-3 minutes.
4. Add cabbage, chopped, and continue frying for 2 minutes more.
5. Add tamari and mix well.
6. Turn off heat, cover and let it rest for 30 seconds.
7. Add Spirulina and enjoy garden fresh vegetables with nature's most perfect food supplement.

Serves 4-8.

SUMMER PEAS PUDDING

3 tbsp. butter or margarine
3 tbsp. flour
¾ cup scalded milk
3 cups fresh or frozen green peas
1 cup water
1 tsp. salt or to taste

2 tbsp. Spirulina
2 tbsp. unflavored gelatin
¼ cup white wine
½ cup chicken, beef or vegetable stock
¾ cup heavy cream
radish roses
parsley

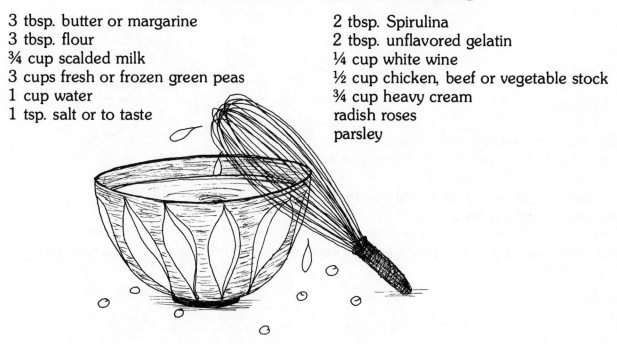

1. In a heavy saucepan melt butter over moderately low heat, stir in the flour and cook the mixture, stirring constantly, for 3 minutes.
2. Remove pan from heat and whisk in the milk.
3. Bring mixture to a boil over moderate heat, whisking, and simmer for another 5 minutes.
4. In another pan combine the peas with the water and salt and bring to a boil, lower heat and simmer for 7 minutes.
5. Drain peas and purée them in blender with milk mixture and Spirulina.
6. Transfer to a bowl and set aside to cool.
7. In a small bowl sprinkle gelatin over the wine to soften.
8. Bring stock to a boil and add the gelatin mixture.
9. Stir until gelatin is dissolved.
10. Add the gelatin mixture into the purée, season with salt and pepper and let it all cool.
11. Meanwhile, beat chilled whipping cream until it holds stiff peaks and fold into the Spirulina/pea purée.
12. You may at this point divide the mixture into six 6-oz. molds rinsed in cold water or into one large mold.
13. Smooth tops and chill puddings.
14. When ready to serve, unmold and garnish with radish roses and parsley and serve with your favorite herbed tomato sauce.

Serves 6.

POTATO NUT LOAF

Richly filling on a cold winter night.

3 cups mashed potato
1 cup ground nuts (pecans, walnuts, peanuts,
    cashews, etc.)
1 cup celery, chopped (including tops)
1 cup grated carrots
1 large onion, chopped
¼ lb. butter
¼ cup fresh chopped parsley

3 tbsp. nutritional yeast
1 tsp. salt or to taste
¼ tsp. nutmeg
¼ tsp. black pepper
1 tbsp. chopped chives
1 tsp. thyme
¼ cup Spirulina
½ lb. sunflower seeds
1 red bell pepper

1. Preheat oven to 350°.
2. Sauté onion in butter.
3. Blend together all the above ingredients, put in oiled baking pan and bake until done—about 35-45 minutes.
4. Garnish with sliced red pepper and serve with Macadamia Nut Sauce.

Macadamia Nut Sauce:

1½ sticks butter
¾ cup sliced Macadamia nuts (you may substitute, but the flavor will not be the same)
¼ cup minced parsley
⅛ cup minced shallots

1. In a heavy skillet melt the butter, add the nuts and cook over low heat until they are golden.
2. Stir in the parsley and shallots.

Makes about 1¼ cups.

Serves 6.

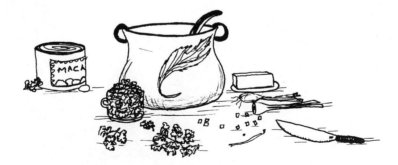

CURD CURRY

Delicious. A very typical vegetarian Indian dish.

Sauce:
1 cup yogurt
¼ cup split pea flour (besan in Indian food
  shops)
1½ tbsp. ghee (clarified butter—see recipe p. 67)
¼ tsp. ginger (freshly chopped or ground)
2 cloves crushed garlic
¼ tsp. turmeric
¼ tsp. black mustard seeds
3 or 4 curry leaves or 1 bay leaf (optional)
½ tsp. ground cumin
¼ tsp. brown sugar
4-5 fenugreek seeds

Spirulina Balls:
1 cup falafel mix
½ tsp. cayenne or to taste
2 tsp. Spirulina
water
oil for deep frying

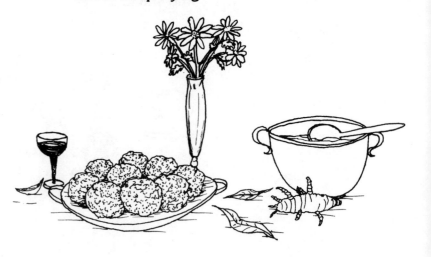

1. Combine yogurt and flour and set aside. A little water may be added if mixture is too thick.
2. Heat ghee in pan and add all remaining sauce ingredients.
3. Sauté 2 minutes.
4. Add the yogurt and flour mixture and let cook on medium flame for 5 minutes.
5. Combine falafel, cayenne and Spirulina together in a bowl.
6. Mix in water to make a stiffish batter.
7. Set aside for a few minutes.
8. Heat the oil in a deep fryer.
9. When hot add the above batter in spoonfuls, lower flame and fry until fritters surface.
10. Remove, drain and then put them into the sauce mixture.
11. Let fritters soak in yogurt mix for at least 1 hour. They will get all puffed up and saturate the curds.

Very nutritious, and now doubly so with the Spirulina added to it. May be eaten plain or with rice or other vegetables.

Serves 4.

CREAMED SPINACH MIMOSA

3 lbs. spinach
6 tbsp. butter
1½-2 cups heavy cream
2 tbsp. Spirulina
dash nutmeg
sieved yolks of 2 hardboiled eggs

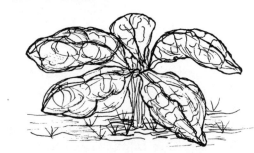

1. Wash spinach well and trim.
2. Cover and cook until tender in a large saucepan with only the water that clings to the washed leaves.
3. Transfer the spinach to a colander and squeeze out as much liquid as possible.
4. Transfer to a cutting board and chop fine.
5. In a large skillet cook spinach in the butter over medium heat, stirring until the moisture has evaporated.
6. Add cream, ½ cup at a time, stirring.
7. Season the spinach with nutmeg, salt and pepper, then simmer over low heat until the cream is reduced to desired consistency.
8. Remove from heat.
9. Mix in Spirulina and transfer the spinach to a heated deep serving dish and decoratively mark it with a metal spatula.
10. Sprinkle the edges with sieved egg yolks.
11. Garnish dish with sautéed croutons and cut in decorative shapes if desired.

Serves 6.

SPINACH, CHEESE AND SPIRULINA QUICHE

2 10 oz. packages frozen spinach
3 tbsp. cream cheese
2 tbsp. sour cream
1 tbsp. Worcestershire sauce
2 tbsp. Spirulina
2 tsp. grated horseradish or 1 tsp. horseradish
   sauce

2 tsp. salt or to taste
1 tsp. basil
1 tsp. pepper
dash of Tabasco
nutmeg to taste
1 pie shell, baked
4 eggs
1½ cups light cream
1 cup grated Gruyère cheese
⅔ cup grated Romano cheese

1. Cook spinach according to directions on package.
2. Refresh under cold running water and squeeze it dry.
3. Set aside.
4. In a bowl combine softened cream cheese, sour cream, Worcestershire sauce, Spirulina, horseradish, salt, basil, pepper, Tabasco and nutmeg.
5. Add the reserved spinach to this mixture and combine thoroughly.
6. Spread evenly in pie shell.
7. In another bowl whisk together 2 whole eggs, 2 egg yolks and the cream. Set aside.
8. Sprinkle the cheeses over the spinach mixture.
9. Put pan on a baking sheet and carefully pour in egg mixture.
10. Bake the quiche in the middle of a preheated moderately hot oven (370°) for 40 minutes or until it is puffed and brown and a knife inserted in center comes out clean.
11. Transfer to a rack and let it cool for 5 minutes.

Serves 6.

STUFFED GREEN PEPPERS

Very delicious and extremely nutritious.

6 green peppers
2 cups brown rice (long or short grain)
2 large onions, diced
1 bunch chopped celery
¾ tsp. Chinese Five Spices (available in Oriental section of supermarket)
3 cloves crushed garlic
½ lb. chopped pastrami (optional)
salt to taste
2 heaped tbsp. Spirulina
¼ tsp. cayenne
1 tsp. coriander powder
2 tbsp. oil
1½-2 qts. tomato sauce
1 tbsp. butter or margarine

1. Cut green peppers in half and seed. Set aside.
2. Boil rice in 3 cups water or vegetable stock.
3. Sauté onions lightly.
4. Add all but last two ingredients and stir fry for a few minutes.
5. Add boiled rice, mix well and taste for seasoning.
6. Add salt as needed.
7. Fill peppers with rice mixture.
8. Put into a baking pan which will hold pepper halves compactly.
9. Pour oil over peppers.
10. Top with tomato sauce.
11. Bake in moderate oven (350°)1½-2 hours.
12. Serve as main course or vegetable.

Serves 12 as a starter or 6 as a main course.

STEWED ASPARAGUS SOUFFLÉ
À LA SPIRULINA

fine bread crumbs
1 can asparagus pieces or ½ lb. fresh
2 tbsp. butter
1½ tbsp. flour
½ cup milk

salt and pepper to taste
1 tbsp. Spirulina
6 eggs
½ cup grated Parmesan cheese
hot melted butter for sauce
1 clove garlic (optional)

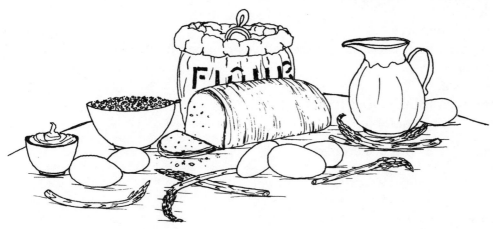

1. Use a round pudding mold 8 inches in diameter that has its own tight-fitting lid (otherwise use foil).
2. Butter the mold well and sprinkle with bread crumbs.
3. Drain the can of asparagus pieces, reserving ½ cup liquid (if using fresh asparagus, boil in salted water, drain and also retain ½ cup liquid).
4. Prepare a thick white sauce with the butter, flour, milk and reserved asparagus liquid.
5. Season with salt and pepper.
6. Whisk in the Spirulina and then add the asparagus pieces.
7. Separate eggs one by one, dropping egg whites into a mixing bowl and dropping egg yolks into the sauce. Stir well after addition of each egg yolk.
8. Beat egg whites until stiff but not dry and fold into the egg yolk mixture.
9. Fill pudding mold with the mixture and cover tightly. (If you do not have a pudding mold with a lid, place a double sheet of foil over the mixture and make sure it is tightly bound with a piece of string; we do not want the water from the steaming pot to leak into the pudding).
10. Set mold into a large saucepan half full of simmering water.
11. Cover saucepan and cook the soufflé on top of the stove for exactly one hour.
12. Turn out and sprinkle with grated cheese.
13. Serve hot with melted butter sauce. (You can sauté the crushed garlic in the sauce to get a garlic butter sauce if you prefer. Discard garlic before serving.)

Serves 6.

SPIRULINA AND PROTEIN

The protein in Spirulina is, on the average, 90% digestible (from 83-95%). Let's compare 100 grams of Spirulina and 100 grams of sirloin steak. Spirulina is 71% protein while meat is about 20% protein, so Spirulina has 71 grams of protein in 100 grams of powder. With 90% usable protein, we are left with 63 grams of usable protein in Spirulina while only 20 grams of protein in 100 grams of meat are available. However, the net protein utilization of beef is roughly 67%, so 20 grams $\times$ 0.67 = 13.4 grams of usable protein in 100 grams of beef.

CHOLESTEROL AND SPIRULINA

The cholesterol sufferer should restrict his diet to less than 300 mg. of cholesterol per day. Three teaspoons of Spirulina give us just 1.4 mg. of cholesterol per day. (See JOURNAL OF NUTRITIONAL MICROBIOLOGY, Vol. 1, No. 10). One egg contains 66 times more cholesterol than 3 teaspoons of Spirulina.

MAIN DISHES—
MEAT, FISH
AND POULTRY

We Ceylonese grow up fondly on fish and so you'll find a generous offering of fish dishes in the following pages. Try the whole gamut—lobster, crab meat, haddock, sole, spiced up with ginger and garlic and green onions—these dishes are fit for the finest of occasions and are protein rich as well.

SAVORY SPIRULINA PUDDING

A delicious and wholesome luncheon dish served with red cabbage salad
with a pungent sweet and sour dressing, hot buttered French bread
and a glass of sparkling wine.

6 tbsp. minced green onion
2 cloves garlic, chopped
½ bunch parsley
4 tbsp. butter or margarine
2 10 oz. packages frozen leaf spinach
1 cup finely shredded dried beef OR
   1 cup best hamburger, lightly sautéed in
   its own fat and drained

¼ cup Spirulina
4 cups ricotta cheese
8 eggs
1½ cups milk
½ tsp. paprika
½ tsp. nutmeg
salt and pepper

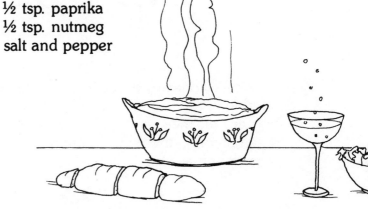

1. In a skillet sauté the onion, garlic and parsley in the butter over moderate heat for 2-3 minutes.
2. Add the spinach which has been defrosted, drained, squeezed and chopped, and sauté mixture for a further 5-6 minutes.
3. Add the beef and Spirulina and cook the mixture for 3 minutes more.
4. Remove from fire.
5. Meanwhile, in a large bowl beat the cheese with the eggs until well combined, add the milk and stir in the spinach/beef mixture.
6. Season well with grated nutmeg, salt and pepper.
7. Pour into a well-buttered 3 quart baking dish.
8. Put dish in a pan, adding enough water to the pan to reach half way up the sides and bake the pudding in a preheated moderately slow oven (325°) for 1½ to 2 hours or until set.

Serves 4-6.

SAVORY SPIRULINA MEAT LOAF

2 lbs. ground beef
2 eggs, slightly beaten
1 large onion, chopped
1 red pepper, chopped
¼ lb. chopped ham
¼ lb. chopped mushrooms
2 bunches parsley, chopped

2 tsp. soy sauce
½ tsp. thyme
¼ tsp. cayenne
2 garlic cloves
2 tbsp. Spirulina
1½ cups whole wheat bread crumbs
salt and pepper to taste
dash of Burgundy

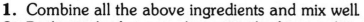

1. Combine all the above ingredients and mix well.
2. Pack into loaf pan or shape into loaf on cookie sheet.
3. Bake in a moderate oven at 350° for 1½ hours.
4. Serve with soy sauce and a dash of Burgundy.

Serves 8-10.

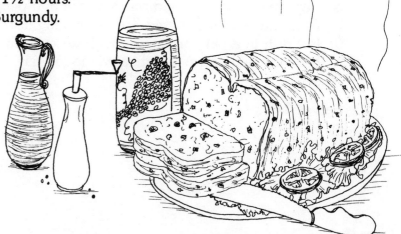

SPICY KEBABS

1½ lbs. ground beef or lamb
1 cup minced onions
1½ tsp. salt or to taste
¼ tsp. ginger
1 tbsp. Spirulina
½ tsp. turmeric
½ tsp. freshly chopped mint
1 tbsp. coriander powder
½ tsp. pepper
1 cup yogurt
¼ cup flour
4 tbsp. butter

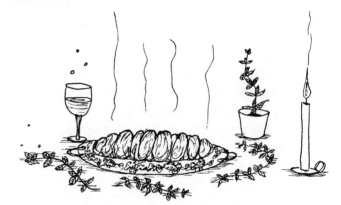

1. Mix together the meat, onions, salt, spices, Spirulina and ½ cup of the yogurt.
2. Roll into sausage shapes 1 inch in diameter and 4 inches in length.
3. Dip in the remaining yogurt and then the flour.
4. Melt the butter in a skillet.
5. Cook the kebabs over low heat until browned on all sides.

Also makes exellent hors d'oeuvres.

Makes about 12 small kebabs.

EMERALD RED PEPPERS

A very good luncheon dish. Served with garlic bread
and a nicely chilled white wine, mmmm.....

6 red bell peppers, cut in half and seeded
1½ lbs. flaked fish (your favorite)
½ bunch chopped parsley
2 sweet gherkins, finely chopped
4 green olives, finely chopped
juice of ½ lemon

pepper, salt, garlic and celery salt to taste
green mayonnaise (recipe follows)
stuffed sliced olives
lemon slices
tomato slices

1. Wash and dry red peppers.
2. Cut in half and seed.
3. Brush with oil and broil for 5 minutes.
4. Set aside to cool.
5. Meanwhile, combine flaked fish with the rest of the ingredients and fold in the green mayonnaise.
6. Chill.
7. Taste for seasonings and adjust accordingly.
8. When ready to serve, pile the mixture into the prepared red pepper shells and garnish with stuffed sliced olives, lemon slices and tomato slices.
9. Serve on a bed of lettuce.

Green Mayonnaise:

1 cup mayonnaise
1 bunch chopped parsley
1 tbsp. snipped chives
½ tbsp. fresh minced tarragon or ¼ tsp. dried
1 tsp. snipped dill
1 tsp. fresh chervil or ¼ tsp. dried
2 tbsp. Spirulina

Combine all the above ingredients well, making sure no Spirulina lumps remain.

GOOD, GOOD, GOOD.

Serves 12 as a starter or 6 as a main course.

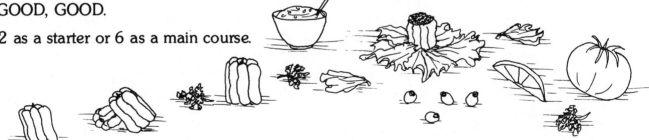

OMELET PRIMAVERA

Three omelets piled high and cut in wedges. Hearty and satisfying.

10 oz. fresh spinach or swiss chard, ribs
    removed
3 anchovy fillets, chopped
1 garlic clove, crushed
6 tbsp. olive or vegetable oil
12 eggs
¼ cup Spirulina

1½ tsp. sea salt
freshly ground pepper
2 tomatoes, peeled, seeded and chopped
1 sweet red pepper, chopped
2 tbsp. onion, chopped
2 tbsp. half and half
½ cup shredded Gruyère cheese

Omelet One:
1. Place spinach with the water that clings to leaves from washing in Dutch oven.
2. Steam, covered, over medium heat until limp, about 2 minutes.
3. Drain and rinse in cold water, pressing out excess moisture in strainer.
4. Sauté anchovies and garlic in 2 tbsp. oil in a 7" skillet over low heat until garlic is golden.
5. Remove anchovies and garlic from skillet.
6. Beat first 4 eggs until light and fluffy and pour into the hot skillet.
7. Chop rinsed spinach and add the Spirulina, anchovies, garlic mixture, ½ tsp. salt and pepper.
8. Add this mixture to the eggs in skillet and cook over low heat until eggs are set. (This takes about 4 minutes.)
9. Invert onto a hot platter and keep warm.

Omelet Two:
10. Heat tomatoes, red pepper and onion in 7" skillet over low heat until liquid evaporates.
11. Add 2 tbsp. oil
12. Beat 4 eggs until light and fluffy and add ½ tsp. salt and pepper.
13. Pour into the tomato mixture.
14. Cook, covered, over low heat until the eggs are set.
15. Invert onto the top of the spinach omelet and keep warm.

Omelet Three:
16. Beat the last 4 eggs until light and fluffy, stir in half and half, ½ tsp. salt and pepper.
17. Heat 2 tbsp. oil in 7" skillet over low heat and pour in egg mixture.
18. Sprinkle with cheese.
19. Cook, covered, over low heat until eggs are set.
20. Invert on top of the other two omelets.
21. Cool to lukewarm.
22. Trim edges and cut into wedges.

Serve with hot whole wheat bread and a green salad...and a glass of vino, too.

Serves 8-10.

STUFFED GRAPE LEAVES
WITH EGG AND LEMON SAUCE

This is a famous Greek dish which is ideal to serve
as finger-food without sauce, or to be dipped in sauce, or as given here
with the sauce poured over the leaves.

1 jar grape leaves, about 40-50
6 oz. ground veal
6 oz. ground beef
⅓ cup chopped fresh dill
6 mint leaves
3 tbsp. grated feta cheese (cheddar may be
  used as a substitute)
⅔ cup cooked rice
2 oz. raisins, chopped

2 tbsp. sunflower seeds
2 tbsp. Spirulina
½ tsp. cinnamon
salt and pepper to taste
2 medium onions, chopped
2 carrots, sliced
2 cups bouillon
1 tbsp. olive oil

1. Carefully remove grape leaves from jar and drain in colander.
2. Combine the veal and beef and mix with all but the last 4 remaining ingredients and one of the onions. Mix well so that all the ingredients are thoroughly combined.
3. Divide the mixture into 40 equal parts.
4. Place 1 part on each of the grape leaves and roll the leaves compactly to enclose the filling completely.
5. Place sliced carrots and remaining onion along the bottom of a saucepan and cover them with 4 or 5 remaining grape leaves.
6. Arrange the stuffed grape leaves in the saucepan and pour the bouillon and olive oil over the stuffed leaves.
7. Heat slowly until liquid begins to boil.
8. Reduce heat and simmer the grape leaves, covered, for 35-40 minutes.
9. Drain and keep warm.

Serves 12.

For sauce recipe see next page.

Sauce:
5 tbsp. flour
½ stick or ¼ cup butter
1½ cups bouillon
1 egg yolk
1 tsp. lemon juice
salt and pepper to taste
milk (optional)

1. In a saucepan over low heat blend flour into the melted butter.
2. Gradually stir in bouillon to form a smooth sauce.
3. Beat in the egg yolk and season the mixture with lemon juice, salt and pepper. (If necessary, thin the sauce with hot milk until it reaches the consistency of heavy cream.)
4. Pour the sauce over the stuffed grape leaves.

TURKEY BALLS

1 lb. ground turkey
3 slices whole wheat bread, crumbed
2 tbsp. finely chopped onion
2 cloves crushed garlic
2 slices ginger, chopped
1 tsp. fennel

½ tsp. powdered cinnamon
½ tsp. cloves
½ tsp. black pepper
salt to taste
½ tsp. red pepper or chili powder
2 eggs
2 tbsp. Spirulina
juice of ½ lime

1. Season the ground turkey with garlic, ginger, fennel, cinnamon, cloves, salt, pepper and chili powder.
2. Add the onions, bread crumbs and Spirulina.
3. Add beaten eggs and lime juice to moisten.
4. Drop by teaspoonfuls into hot oil and fry until golden.

Serve with sweet and sour sauce.

Makes about 50-60.

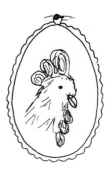

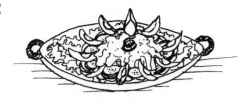

EGGS IN SPIRULINA/PARSLEY SAUCE

1 cup parsley sprigs
12 pitted green olives
1 clove crushed garlic
1 tbsp. capers

3 anchovy fillets, rinsed and patted dry
½ cup olive oil or vegetable oil
2 tbsp. Spirulina
6 hardboiled eggs, sliced
cucumber twist

1. In a blender or food processor purée the parsley, olives, garlic, capers and anchovy fillets.
2. Add the oil in a stream.
3. Add the Spirulina.
4. Arrange egg slices on a serving platter and pour sauce over them, or serve on individual platters by slicing the egg and layering on a bed of finely sliced cucumbers and then pouring the sauce over.
5. Garnish with a cucumber twist.

Serves 6.

HADDOCK AND RICE MOLD

Good for a ladies' luncheon, a brunch or a late after theatre
light supper dish, or whenever you like something a bit extra special.

Rice Mixture:
1½ cups long grain white rice (preferably a good quality Indian or Persian)
3 tbsp. salt
2 tbsp. butter
⅓ cup minced onion
⅓ cup minced carrots
⅓ cup minced celery
salt and pepper to taste
3 tbsp. Spirulina
½ tsp. thyme

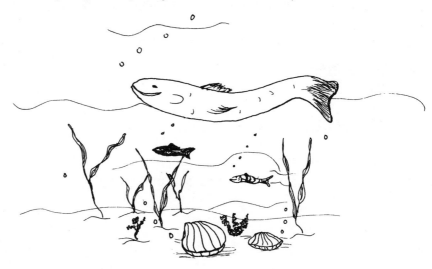

1. Wash rice under running cold water until water runs clear. Transfer rice to a bowl.
2. Add salt and enough cold water to cover by 1 inch and leave to soak overnight.
3. Drain rice and reserve.
4. In a skillet heat butter, add the onions, carrots, celery, thyme, salt and pepper and steam the vegetables, covered with a buttered round of wax paper and the lid, over moderately low heat for 10 minutes or until they are tender.
5. Add Spirulina and stir in gently but thoroughly.
6. Transfer to a bowl and keep covered.

Haddock Mixture:
3½ lbs. haddock fillets
salt and pepper
1½ cups white fish stock
¾ cup milk
½ cup heavy cream
seasonings (your favorite herbs, salt and pepper)
lemon slices

1. Halve the haddock fillets lengthwise.
2. Cut each fillet in half crosswise and flatten the pieces between wax paper.
3. Sprinkle fish with salt and pepper, spread about 1 tbsp. vegetable mixture on each piece of fish and roll tightly.
4. Butter a 1½ quart round glass dish generously with softened butter and spread half the reserved rice in the dish.
5. Brush the fish rolls with melted butter and stand them on the rice.
6. In a saucepan combine 1 cup of the fish stock (reserve ½ cup), milk and cream and bring the liquid to a boil and pour it over the rolls.
7. Spread the remaining rice over the rolls and dot it with softened butter.
8. Heat a baking tray on the lowest rack of a preheated oven (420°) for 5 minutes and bake the mixture on the sheet for 25 minutes.
9. Bake it, covered with a buttered round of wax paper, for 15 minutes more.
10. In a saucepan bring the remaining fish stock to a boil, pour it over the rice mixture and bake the mixture, covered with a wax paper for a further 20 minutes or until golden brown.
11. Let the dish stand at room temperature for 5 minutes.
12. Run a metal spatula around the inside of the mold, invert a heated serving dish over the mold, and invert the mold onto the dish.
13. Garnish the dish with thin slices of lemon and serve with a white wine sauce for fish.

Serve with ice cold cucumber and dill salad.

Serves 6-8.

SWEET AND SOUR FISH

1 cucumber
1 carrot
1 sweet pickle
1 tsp. chopped ginger
½ cup minced onion
salt to taste
2 tbsp. honey
½ cup vinegar
½ cup water

4 tbsp. oil
1 carp or snapper (3 lbs.), or fillets if a whole
    fish is unavailable
1 tbsp. cornstarch
1 tbsp. soy sauce
2 minced garlic cloves
1 tbsp. Spirulina
parsley
lemon slices

1. Pare the cucumbers and cut in half lengthwise.
2. Scoop out the seeds and cut into fine slices.
3. Cut carrot in same size pieces.
4. Slice pickle.
5. Combine the previous ingredients with the ginger, onion, salt, honey, vinegar and water.
6. Let marinate ¾ hour.

If using whole fish (which has been cleaned):

7. Bring 2 quarts of water to a boil.
8. Add salt to taste and 2 tbsp. of the oil.
9. Carefully place fish in the skillet.
10. Cover and cook over low heat and let fish cook until tender. Proceed to Step 14.

If using sliced fish:

11. Dust fish in seasoning, salt, pepper and lemon juice.
12. Layer fish in baking pan and pour over it 2 tbsp. oil.
13. Put in preheated oven and bake for 20 minutes at 350°. (This should be done preferably in one layer.)
14. Drain the vegetables.
15. Mix the marinade with the cornstarch and soy sauce.
16. Heat the remaining 2 tbsp. oil in a skillet and brown the garlic in it.
17. Add the marinade, stirring constantly.
18. Add vegetables and just let them heat, but don't cook them.
19. Remove from fire and stir in the Spirulina.
20. Carefully place fish on a platter.
21. Pour sauce over it.
22. Garnish with parsley and lemon slices.

Serves 4-6.

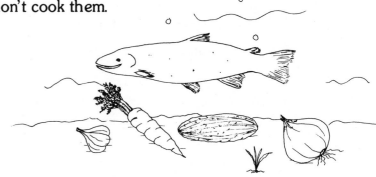

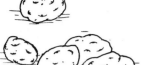

ANCHOVY STUFFED TOMATOES

Red tomato with just a hint of green around the rim
and the pale cream potato nestling in the center.

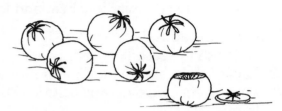

6 tomatoes
¼ can chopped anchovies
1½ tsp. Spirulina
⅛ tsp. cayenne
1½ lbs. potatoes (boiled and mashed with butter)

1. Slice tops of tomatoes, scoop out center and place upside down on paper towels to drain.
2. Mix well the anchovies (with oil from can), Spirulina, cayenne, and ½ of the scooped out tomato, chopped small.
3. Put ½ tsp. of this mixture at the bottom of each tomato.
4. Fill a cake decorator bag with mashed potatoes and fill the tomato shell, forming a rosette.
5. Bake in a moderate oven (350°) for about ½-¾ hour.

This dish is quite delightful to see.

Serves 6.

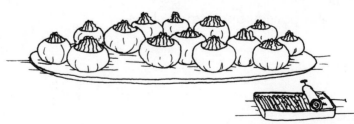

SEAFOOD EXTRAVAGANZA

1⅓ cups minced onion
½ stick butter or margarine
1 cup long grain rice (brown or white)
½ cup minced parsley
¾ tsp. thyme
2 garlic cloves, minced
½ tsp. fennel
1 tsp. Lawry's Salt

½ tsp. black pepper
2 cups fish or chicken stock
½ lb. shelled and deveined shrimp
½ pt. shucked oysters
¼ lb. flaked crab meat
½ stick butter or margarine
1 tbsp. cognac or 2-3 tbsp. sherry
2 tbsp. Spirulina

1. In a flame-proof casserole dish sauté onion in the butter over medium heat for about 10 minutes.
2. Add rice and cook, stirring, for about 5 minutes or until rice is golden.
3. Stir in the parsley, thyme, garlic cloves, fennel, Lawry's Salt and black pepper.
4. Mix well.
5. Add stock.
6. Bring liquid to a boil.
7. Remove from flame and bake in a preheated oven (350°) for 25-30 minutes or until the liquid is absorbed.
8. In a skillet sauté shrimp, oysters and crab meat in the butter for 1-2 minutes.
9. Add cognac or sherry.
10. Toss well.
11. Add the seafood and Spirulina to the rice mixture and serve with poultry or a plain salad and fish.

Serves 4.

SPIRULINA/EGG, SALMON RIBBON LOAF

A work of art in yellow/pink pastels!

1 loaf unsliced sandwich bread or whole wheat bread
4-6 oz. butter or margarine, softened
1 cup salmon spread (recipe follows)
1 tomato, peeled and thinly sliced
1 cup egg salad spread (recipe follows)
⅓ cup milk
12 oz. cream cheese, softened
parsley
1 bunch radishes, sliced, or radish roses

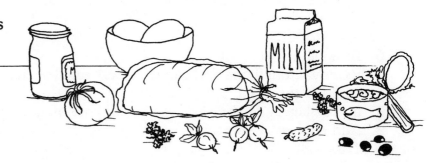

1. Dust tomato in salt and pepper and drain.
2. Trim crusts from bread.
3. Slice lengthwise into 4 layers and butter layers.
4. Spread first layer of bread with salmon spread.
5. Put a layer of buttered bread on top of salmon spread and arrange the sliced tomato on second layer.
6. Place third slice of bread over tomato and spread egg salad spread on it.
7. Top with fourth slice of bread.
8. Transfer the loaf onto a large sheet of foil and chill well.
9. Pour milk into blender, and while it is running, slowly add softened cream cheese.
10. Blend till fluffy.
11. Frost loaf with mixture.
12. Chill till firm.
13. Garnish with parsley and radish slices.

Makes 10 slices.

For Spread recipes see next page.

Salmon Spread:
¼ cup mayonnaise
1 tsp. lemon juice
7¾ oz. can salmon, drained
¼ cup pitted black olives
½ stalk celery
½ tsp. prepared horseradish

Blend all above ingredients in blender till olives and celery are chopped.

Makes 1 cup.

Egg Salad Spread:
¼ cup mayonnaise
4 hardcooked eggs
1 tbsp. Spirulina
1 large sweet pickle
1 green onion, chopped, stocks included
¼ red pepper, sliced
salt and pepper to taste

Blend all above ingredients in blender till mixture is well combined.

Makes 1 cup.

SALMON MOUSSE

1 pkg. unflavored gelatin
¼ cup cold water
½ cup boiling water
½ cup mayonnaise
1 tbsp. lemon juice
1 tbsp. grated onion
½ tsp. Tabasco sauce

1 tsp. salt
1½ tsp. Spirulina
1 can red salmon (15½ oz., or half salmon
   and half crab meat)
½ cup heavy cream, whipped
cucumber swirls
tomato aspic flowers

1. In a large bowl sprinkle gelatin over cold water to soften.
2. Add boiling water and stir until dissolved. Let cool about 5 minutes.
3. Add mayonnaise, lemon juice, onion, Tabasco sauce, salt and Spirulina. Mix well until thoroughly blended.
4. Chill until the consistency of egg white is reached.
5. Drain salmon and flake or purée in blender.
6. Fold into gelatin mixture.
7. Gently fold whipped cream into salmon mixture.
8. Turn into a 4 cup decorative mold and refrigerate until firm, about 4 hours or overnight.
9. Remove from mold and garnish with cucumber swirls and tomato aspic flowers.

Delicious as a main course or to be served with crackers as an appetizer.

Serves 8.

SALMON SPINACH SOUFFLÉ

Spinach Mixture:
2 lbs. spinach (mustard greens or chard may
     be used)
3 tbsp. butter
½ cup béchamel sauce
2 tbsp. heavy cream
2 tbsp. Spirulina
salt and pepper to taste

Salmon Mixture:
2 tbsp. minced onion
3 tbsp. butter
5 tbsp. flour
1¼ cups milk, scalded
4 eggs, separated
1½ cups cooked flaked salmon
1 tbsp. tomato paste
cayenne, salt and pepper to taste

1. Lightly butter a 1½ quart soufflé dish. Set aside.
2. In a skillet sauté the trimmed, washed, squeezed dry spinach in the butter for 5 minutes, or until moisture has evaporated.
3. Add the béchamel sauce, cream, Spirulina and salt and pepper. Set aside.
4. Sauté onion in the butter until it is softened.
5. Add flour and cook the mixture over low heat, stirring, for 2 minutes.
6. Remove pan from heat, add the scalded milk in a stream, whisking, and cook the sauce over moderate heat, stirring constantly, until it is thickened.
7. Remove pan from heat and add the egg yolks, 1 at a time, beating well after each addition.
8. Stir in the flaked salmon, tomato paste, cayenne and salt and pepper.
9. In another bowl beat the egg whites until they hold stiff peaks, fold ⅓ of the whites into the salmon mixture, and fold the mixture into the remaining whites.
10. Arrange spinach mixture in the bottom of the soufflé dish and pour the salmon mixture over it.
11. Bake the soufflé in the middle of a preheated oven (370°) for 45 minutes, or until it is puffed and golden.

Serves 6-8.

BAKED CLAMS A LA SPIRULINA

De-elicious.

3 7½ oz. cans minced clams
bottled clam juice
1 tbsp. cornstarch
1 tbsp. soy sauce
dash cayenne
¼ cup green onions, minced
1 cup tiny green peas, cooked, fresh or frozen
1 cup corn
¼ cup water chestnuts, chopped
1 tbsp. Spirulina
tomato slices

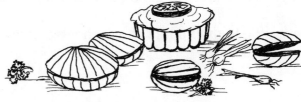

1. Drain the clams and measure the juice.
2. Add enough bottled clam juice to make 1 cup.
3. Mix together the cornstarch, soy sauce and clam juice.
4. Cook over low heat, stirring constantly until thickened.
5. Add cayenne.
6. Stir in the green onions, peas, corn, water chestnuts, Spirulina and clams.
7. Divide among 8 individual soufflé dishes.
8. Top each with a slice of tomato.
9. Put under preheated broiler for 5 minutes.

You may serve it in one big Pyrex or Corning Ware dish instead of individual dishes.

Serves 8.

LOBSTER STRUDEL

Sauce:
½ stick butter (2 oz.)
3 tbsp. flour
1 cup milk, scalded
⅓ cup grated Gruyère cheese
2 tbsp. heavy cream
¼ tsp. dry mustard
2 tbsp. Spirulina
salt and pepper to taste
2 tbsp. cognac (optional)

1. In a saucepan melt the butter, stir in the flour and cook the mixture over low heat, stirring for 3 minutes.
2. Remove pan from heat and add the scalded milk in a stream, whisking vigorously until the mixture is thick and smooth.
3. Simmer the sauce for 5 minutes.
4. Stir in cheese, cream, mustard, Spirulina, salt and pepper and cognac.
5. Stir well and leave to cool, covered with a round of buttered wax paper. (This prevents a skin from forming.)

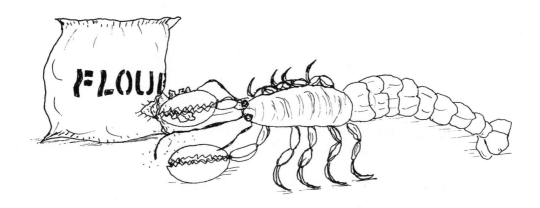

Fish Mixture:
2 cups chopped cooked lobster meat
1 cup cooked chopped shrimp
1 cup cooked chopped sole or flounder
½ cup chopped mushrooms, sautéed in 2 tbsp. butter

*Phyllo leaves:
15 phyllo leaves (available in specialty grocery stores)
1½ sticks butter, melted
¾ cup stale bread crumbs

*To make life easier you could use frozen puff pastry instead of phyllo leaves.

1. Add sauce to the fish mixture and combine carefully.
2. Have ready the 15 phyllo leaves and melted butter.
3. Brush 3 leaves with butter, sprinkle the buttered leaves with stale bread crumbs, and stack them.
4. Spread a strip of the seafood/Spirulina mixture (about ¾ cup) 1 inch from the edge of one of the long sides of the buttered phyllo, fold in the sides of the leaves to contain the mixture, and roll up the leaves jellyroll fashion.
5. Continue to make rolls with the remaining phyllo, butter, bread crumbs and filling in the same manner.
6. Transfer the rolls to buttered baking sheets seam side down, brush the tops with melted butter, and bake the rolls in a preheated moderate oven (350°) for 40-45 minutes, or until they are crisp and golden.
7. Let the strudel cool for 5 minutes and cut each roll into 4 pieces.

Serves 20 as a first course.

SPINACH ROLL WITH CRAB MEAT STUFFING

Very tasty served with salad and pasta.

Spinach Roll:
3 lbs. spinach or 3 10 oz. packets frozen leaf
   spinach
⅓ cup minced onion
6 tbsp. butter
¼ cup heavy cream
¼ tsp. nutmeg
salt and pepper to taste
5 eggs, separated
1½ tbsp. Spirulina

Filling:
1 lb. shredded crab meat
½ cup snipped chives
1 tbsp. butter
1 cup grated carrots
cayenne to taste
1 tsp. lemon juice or to taste
2 cloves minced garlic
melted butter
bread crumbs

1. Cook the fresh or frozen spinach in a kettle until tender.
2. Drain the spinach in a colander and refresh under cold running water until it is cool.
3. Squeeze the spinach well and chop it coarsely.
4. In a skillet sauté onion in the butter until it is lightly colored, add spinach and cook for 3-4 minutes or until the spinach and onion are well combined and coated with the butter.
5. Add cream and cook the mixture, stirring, until the cream is absorbed.
6. Season spinach mixture with nutmeg, salt and pepper to taste.
7. Transfer to a large bowl and beat in the 5 egg yolks, 1 at a time.
8. Whisk in Spirulina.
9. Line a buttered 15½ inch by 10½ inch jellyroll pan with wax paper and butter the paper well.
10. Beat the egg whites with a pinch of salt until they hold stiff peaks.
11. Stir ¼ of the whites into the spinach mixture and fold in the remaining whites, and spread the mixture in the pan.
12. Bake the spinach mixture in a preheated moderate oven (350°) for 20-25 minutes, or until it is firm.
13. Cover the spinach soufflé with a tea towel and a baking sheet and invert it onto the sheet.
14. Remove the wax paper and with the long side across, roll the spinach soufflé in the towel jellyroll fashion.
15. Let the soufflé cool*, unroll it and spread it with the crab mixture.
16. Reroll the soufflé and chill it, wrapped in foil, for at least 1 hour.
17. Slice the roll into 1-inch slices and arrange the slices in a well-buttered oven proof dish.
18. Sprinkle the slices with melted butter and bread crumbs and bake them, covered with foil, in a preheated oven (375°) for 25 minutes or until hot.

This dish may be served cold as well, whichever you prefer. I have found this to be a convenient dish to make as I can assemble it the day before and refrigerate, deciding on the day it is to be served whether I want to serve it hot or cold.

*You may, however, spread the crab mixture immediately after it is taken out of the jellyroll pan and follow the same procedure.

Serve hot with sauce boat of melted butter.

Serves 6-8.

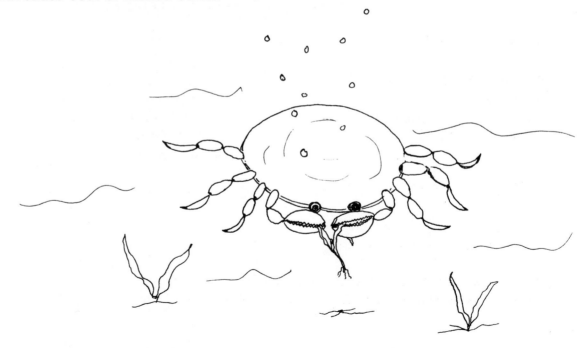

1. In 12 inch skillet over medium-high heat, melt 3 tbsp. butter or margarine.
2. Add chicken and cook until browned on all sides.
3. Add water, pepper and bouillon.
4. Heat to boiling.
5. Reduce heat to low, cover, simmer 30 minutes or until fork-tender.
6. Meanwhile, with sharp knife, cut 1 lemon crosswise into thin slices, cut each slice in half and set aside for garnish later.
7. Squeeze remaining lemon to make 1 tbsp. juice.
8. In 4 quart saucepan over medium heat, melt 2 tbsp. butter or margarine.
9. Add lemon juice, mushrooms and salt and cook until mushrooms are tender, stirring occasionally.
10. With slotted spoon, spoon mushrooms into small bowl.
11. Add spinach to liquid remaining in saucepan and cook over high heat just until wilted, 2 to 3 minutes, stirring occasionally.
12. Stir in mushrooms.
13. Add Spirulina and keep warm.
14. Skim off fat from liquid in skillet.
15. In cup, mix milk and flour and gradually stir mixture and horseradish into liquid in skillet.
16. Add sunflower seeds and cook over medium heat until slightly thickened, stirring constantly.
17. To serve, arrange spinach mixture on platter and top with chicken pieces. Garnish with reserved lemon slices.

Pass gravy to spoon over chicken and spinach.

Serves 4.

MANICOTTI WITH CHICKEN
AND SPINACH STUFFING

Very delicious and satisfying dish served with a crisp salad,
a heady red wine (or to your taste) and homemade bread to mop up the rich sauce.

½ cup minced onion
¼ cup butter or oil
1 cup cooked and strained spinach
salt and pepper to taste
½ tsp. grated nutmeg
2 cups minced cooked chicken (or turkey)

1 cup ricotta cheese
¼ cup freshly grated Parmesan cheese
⅔ cup whipping cream
¼ cup minced parsley
2 tbsp. Spirulina
2 boxes manicotti for stuffing (8 shells to a box)
8 cups of your favorite mushroom sauce, or a combination of mushroom sauce and white sauce or mushroom and tomato sauce

1. In a heavy skillet sauté the onions in the butter or oil until the onion is softened or lightly browned.
2. Stir in the spinach, combining it well with all the other ingredients (except the sauce).
3. Make sure the Spirulina is well mixed in.
4. Fill the uncooked shells with the above mixture and set aside.
5. Cover the bottom of a baking pan with 2 cups of the sauce and arrange the shells over this sauce in a single layer.
6. Leave some space between each shell so there may be room for expansion in the cooking process.
7. If there is any filling left over it can be mixed in with the remaining sauce and then poured over the shells, covering them completely.
8. Cover dish with foil and bake at 375° for about 1 hour.

Serves 8.

CHICKEN-SPINACH QUICHE

piecrust mix for 9 in. piecrust
3 tbsp. butter or margarine
1 green onion, minced
2 cups half and half
1 teaspoon salt
⅛ tsp. pepper

3 eggs
¼ lb. Swiss cheese, shredded
10 oz. pkg. frozen chopped spinach or kale,
    thawed and squeezed dry
7 oz. cooked chicken, chopped
1 tbsp. Spirulina

1. Prepare piecrust mix as label directs and line 9 inch pie plate.
2. Spread crust with 1 tbsp. softened butter or margarine.
3. Melt 2 tbsp. butter or margarine in 1 quart saucepan over medium heat.
4. Add green onion and cook until tender, stirring occasionally.
5. Remove saucepan from heat. Set aside.
6. In medium bowl with wire whisk or fork mix half and half, salt, pepper, eggs and Spirulina.
7. Stir in cheese, spinach, chicken and green onion mixture and pour into piecrust.
8. Bake 15 minutes in preheated 425° oven and then turn oven control to 325°.
9. Bake 30 minutes longer or until knife inserted in center comes out clean.

Serves 6.

ROLL CUTLETS

1 lb. mashed potatoes
1 lb. salmon, haddock or halibut, boiled
1 tbsp. chopped green onion
1 tbsp. chopped fennel
salt and black pepper to taste

⅛ tsp. powdered cloves
⅛ tsp. garlic powder
juice of 1 lemon
1 tbsp. Spirulina
2 eggs, lightly beaten
1 lb. bread crumbs

1. Boil potatoes, mash and set aside.
2. Mash boiled fish, making sure there are no bones.
3. Add all but last 2 ingredients and mix well so that all the flavors are incorporated.
4. Divide the mashed potato into 10-12 portions.
5. Divide the fish into 10-12 portions.
6. Take one portion of mashed potato and flatten until about ¾ inch thick.
7. Place a portion of fish in the center. Mound the potato around the Spirulina/fish mixture, keeping the cutlets in a long roll shape.
8. Beat the eggs and dip the cutlets in the beaten egg, then coat them thickly with the bread crumbs.
9. Deep fry until golden brown.

Delicious served with warm chili or tomato sauce.

Serves 6.

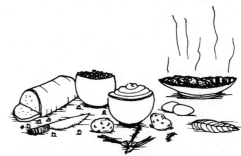

CHICKEN CUTLETS PAPRIKA

1 medium carrot
1 cup water
2 whole large chicken breasts
3 tbsp. flour
salt

salad oil
butter or margarine
1 green onion, thinly sliced
1½ tsp. paprika
1 cup half and half
1 tbsp. Spirulina

1. Prepare garnish: thinly slice carrot. With ½ inch flower-shaped canape cutter, cut carrot slices to resemble flower petals.
2. In 1 quart saucepan over high heat, heat water to boiling.
3. Add carrot flowers; cook about 3 minutes or until carrots are tender.
4. Drain and set aside.
5. On cutting board, cut each chicken breast in half. Working with one half at a time, place it skin-side up.
6. With tip of sharp knife, starting parallel and close to large end of rib bone, cut and scrape meat away from bone and rib cage, gently pulling back meat in one piece as you cut.
7. Discard bones and skin and cut off white tendon.
8. Holding knife parallel to work surface, slice each piece of boneless breast horizontally in half to make 2 cutlets.
9. With meat mallet or dull edge of French knife, pound each chicken cutlet to about ⅛" thickness.

10. On waxed paper, mix flour and 1 teaspoon salt. Coat chicken cutlets with flour mixture.
11. In 12-inch skillet over medium high heat, in 1 tablespoon hot salad oil and 1 tablespoon butter or margine, cook half of chicken cutlets at a time until lightly browned on both sides, about 1 minute, adding more salad oil and butter or margarine if necessary.
12. Remove chicken cutlets to plate; keep warm.
13. Reduce heat to medium.
14. In drippings in skillet, cook green onion until almost tender, stirring occasionally.
15. Stir in paprika; cook 1 minute.
16. Add half and half and ½ teaspoon salt, scraping to loosen brown bits from bottom of skillet.
17. Cook 3 minutes or until slightly thickened, stirring frequently.
18. Stir in Spirulina and whisk till smooth and incorporated well into sauce.
19. Return chicken to a separate skillet and warm through.
20. To serve, arrange chicken on a deep warm platter and spoon sauce over it. Garnish with carrot flowers.

Serves 4.

CHEMICAL ANALYSIS OF SPIRULINA*

CHEMICAL COMPOSITION

Moisture	7.0%
Ash	9.0%
Proteins	71.0%
Crude fiber	0.9%
Xanthophylls	1.80 g/kg of product
Carotene	1.90 g/kg of product
Chlorophyll a	7.60 g/kg of product

TOTAL ORGANIC NITROGEN 13.35%

Nitrogen from Proteins	11.36%
Crude Protein (%N x 6.25)	71.0%

ESSENTIAL AMINOACIDS

Isoleucine	4.13%
Leucine	5.80%
Lysine	4.00%
Methionine	2.17%
Phenylalanine	3.95%
Threonine	4.17%
Tryptophan	1.13%
Valine	6.00%

NON-ESSENTIAL AMINOACIDS

Alanine	5.82%
Arginine	5.98%
Aspartic Acid	6.43%
Cystine	0.67%
Glutamic Acid	8.94%
Glycine	3.46%
Histidine	1.08%
Proline	2.97%
Serine	4.00%
Tyrosine	4.60%

VITAMINS

Biotin (H)	average	0.4	mg/kg
Cyanocobalamin (B_{12})	average	2	mg/kg
d-Ca-Pantothenate	average	11	mg/kg
Folic Acid	average	0.5	mg/kg
Inositol	average	350	mg/kg
Nicotinic Acid (PP)	average	118	mg/kg
Pyridoxine (B_6)	average	3	mg/kg
Riboflavine (B_2)	average	40	mg/kg
Thiamine (B_1)	average	55	mg/kg
Tocopherol (E)	average	190	mg/kg

MOISTURE 7.0%

ASH 9.0%

Calcium (Ca)	1,315	mg/kg
Phosphorus (P)	8,942	mg/kg
Iron (Fe)	580	mg/kg
Sodium (Na)	412	mg/kg
Chloride (Cl)	4,400	mg/kg
Magnesium (Mg)	1,915	mg/kg
Manganese (Mn)	25	mg/kg
Zinc (Zn)	39	mg/kg
Potassium (K)	15,400	mg/kg
Others	57,000	mg/kg

STEROLS

Cholesterol	325	mg/kg
Sitosterol	196	mg/kg
	97	mg/kg
Dihidro 7 Cholesterol } Cholesten 7 ol 3 } — Stigmasterol } others }	32	mg/kg

NUTRITIONAL VALUE

Protein Efficiency Ratio (PER) of 2.2 to 2.6 (74-87% that of casein)
Net Protein Utilization (NPU) of 53 to 61% (85-92% that of casein)
Digestibility of 83 to 84%

Available Lysine	average	85%

NITROGEN FROM NUCLEIC ACIDS 1.99%

Ribonucleic Acid (RNA) RNA = N × 2.18	3.50%
Deoxyribonucleic Acid (DNA) DNA = N × 2.63	1.00%

CAROTENOIDS 4,000 mg/kg

α Carotene	average	traces	mg/kg
β Carotene	average	1,700	mg/kg
Xanthophylis	average	1,000	mg/kg
Cryptoxanthin	average	556	mg/kg
Echinenone	average	439	mg/kg
Zeaxanthin	average	316	mg/kg
Lutein and Euglenanone	average	289	mg/kg

TOTAL LIPIDS 7.0%

Fatty Acids 5.7%

Lauric (C_{12})	229	mg/kg
Myristic (C_{14})	644	mg/kg
Palmitic (C_{16})	21,141	mg/kg
Palmitoleic (C_{16})	2,035	mg/kg
Palmitolinoleic (C_{16})	2,565	mg/kg
Heptadecanoic (C_{17})	142	mg/kg
Stearic (C_{18})	353	mg/kg
Oleic (C_{18})	3,009	mg/kg
γ Linolenic (C_{18})	13,784	mg/kg
Linoleic (C_{18})	11,970	mg/kg
α Linolenic (C_{18})	427	mg/kg
Others	699	mg/kg

Insaponifiable 1.3%

Sterols	325	mg/kg
Titerpen alcohols	800	mg/kg
Carotenoids	4,000	mg/kg
Chlorophyll a	7,600	mg/kg
Others	150	mg/kg
3-4 Benzpyrene	3.6	mg/kg

TOTAL CARBOHYDRATES 16.5%

Ramnose	average	9.0%
Glucane	average	1.5%
Phosphoryled cyclitols	average	2.5%
Glucosamine and muramic acid	average	2.0%
Glycogen	average	0.5%
Sialic acid and others	average	0.5%

* United Nations Laboratories analysis in Holland. The Japanese analysis lists protein digestibility at 95.1%.

SALADS

A huge, fresh, multi-colored salad topped with Spirulina dressing and crunchy nuts or sesame seeds can be the crowning touch of any gourmet meal. Make sure the vegetables are chilled and crisp. On a hot summer afternoon many of these recipes are totally satisfying as meals in themselves. Use your creativity in combining them with the dressings listed in the next section.

BEAN SPROUT SALAD

1 tsp. honey
¼ cup oil
2 tbsp. vinegar
2 tbsp. soy sauce
½ tsp. salt
½ tsp. freshly ground black pepper

¼ cup finely chopped green onions
¼ cup pimento, cut in strips
2 tbsp. ground sesame seeds
1 clove minced garlic
½ tbsp. Spirulina
2 cups bean sprouts

1. Mix together the honey, oil, vinegar, soy sauce, salt, pepper, green onions, pimento, sesame seeds, garlic and Spirulina.
2. Pour over the sprouts and toss lightly.
3. Chill 1 hour.

Serves 4-6.

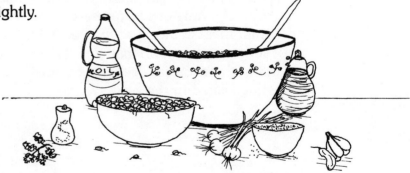

LETTUCE SALAD WITH
SPIRULINA HONEY CREAM DRESSING

About ⅔ lb. leaf lettuce
¼ cup whipping cream
2 tsp. honey
2 tsp. vinegar

½ tbsp. Spirulina
⅛ tsp. salt or to taste
½ tsp. pepper
1 tbsp. chopped chives
4-5 radishes, finely sliced

1. Tear lettuce and place in salad bowl.
2. Place cream, honey, vinegar, Spirulina, salt and pepper in a jar with screw top lid and shake mixture well.
3. Pour Spirulina dressing over salad leaves.
4. Toss gently.
5. Garnish with chopped chives and sliced radishes.

Serves 4.

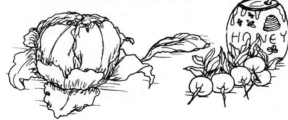

BUCKWHEAT SALAD

Quite, quite delicious and refreshing.

Salad:
1½ cups cooked buckwheat groats or bulgar
½ cup each of minced parsley and dill
⅓ cup chopped red pepper
⅓ cup chopped green onion
5-6 radishes, thinly sliced
salt and pepper to taste

Dressing:
2 tbsp. each olive oil and vegetable oil
1 tbsp. rice wine vinegar (available in Orien-
    tal section of supermarket)
2 tsp. Dijon mustard
1½ tsp. minced garlic
salt and pepper to taste
1½ tsp. warm honey
1 tbsp. Spirulina
6 hard boiled eggs
1 can black olives
1 tomato, cut in wedges

1. Combine the first six ingredients in a bowl.
2. In another bowl or screw-top jar combine the dressing ingredients and shake well. (Must be well combined.)
3. Stir the dressing into the buckwheat mixture and combine well.
4. Chill the salad for at least 30-40 minutes.
5. Line a serving tray with lettuce and serve the salad on it (or if you wish you may serve on individual salad plates on a lettuce leaf).
6. Garnish with quartered eggs, tomato wedges and black olives.

Serves 6.

CHICKEN SALAD

Flavored with a pungent marinade.

1 fryer chicken (3½ lbs.)
½ cup dry sherry
½ cup soy sauce
1 tsp. honey
¼ tsp. cayenne or to taste
¼ tsp. ginger powder
2 garlic cloves, crushed
3 tbsp. oil

2 cups shredded lettuce
¾ cup diced celery
¾ cup bean sprouts
2 tbsp. sesame seeds
1 bunch green onions, finely sliced
½ cup blanched chopped almonds
1 tbsp. Spirulina

1. Cut the chicken from the bone and into bite-size pieces.
2. Marinate for 3 hours in a mixture of sherry, soy sauce, honey, cayenne, ginger and garlic.
3. Drain and reserve the marinade.
4. Heat the oil in a skillet and brown the chicken in it.
5. Cover and cook over low heat for 10 minutes, or until chicken is tender.
6. Cool.
7. Mix together the lettuce, celery, bean sprouts, sesame seeds, green onions, chicken and almonds.
8. Meanwhile, lightly warm the marinade over low heat for 2-3 minutes.
9. Remove from fire and add Spirulina which has been mixed to a paste with ½ cup water.
10. Cool.
11. Mix with the chicken salad and serve cold.

Serves 4-6.

CUCUMBER SPIRULINA SALAD

1 large cucumber, peeled if waxed, otherwise leave unpeeled
3 oz. packet lime flavored gelatin
1 tbsp. Spirulina
1¼ cups boiling water
carrot curls

1. Halve cucumber lengthwise and remove seeds, if desired.
2. Cut in quarters, place in blender and blend till puréed.
3. Measure cucumber and add water if necessary to make a cup.
4. Dissolve gelatin in boiling water, add to puréed cucumber and leave to cool.
5. Whisk in Spirulina and chill until partially set.
6. Pour into 3½ cup mold and chill till set.
7. Unmold the salad and surround wtih carrot curls, or if you are using a ring mold fill the center with the carrot curls.
8. Serve with cottage cheese dressing.

Cottage Cheese Dressing:

1¼ cups cream style cottage cheese
2½ tbsp. honey
5 tsp. lemon juice
2½ tbsp. milk
salt to taste

1. Put cottage cheese, honey, lemon juice and salt in blender.
2. Blend till mixture is creamy.
3. Add milk a tablespoon at a time and blend till desired consistency is reached.

This dressing is delicious on other green leafy type salads as well.

Serves 6-8.

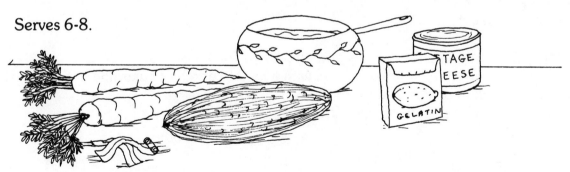

MIXED GREEN SALAD
WITH SPIRULINA CREAM DRESSING

1 head Boston lettuce
1 head red leaf lettuce
1 head curly chicory
1 head romaine
1 head escarole
½ avocado, cubed
½ cucumber (unwaxed)

1. Tear the greens into bite-size pieces and chill them for 1 hour.
2. Combine the greens in a large salad bowl with avocado and half cucumber, scored with the tines of a fork and sliced paper thin.
3. Toss the salad with Spirulina Cream Dressing.

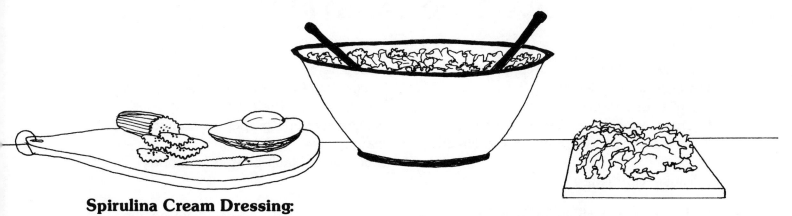

Spirulina Cream Dressing:

½ cup cream
⅓ cup ripe avocado, cubed
⅓ cup cucumber, cubed
1 tbsp. Spirulina

3 tbsp. lemon juice
2 tbsp. minced green onion
½ tsp. minced garlic (to taste)
½ tsp. salt (to taste)
½ tsp. pepper (to taste)

Blend all ingredients in a food processor until smooth and light.

Serves 8-10.

AVOCADO SALAD RING

Makes a delicious decorative mold.

3 oz. packet lemon flavored gelatin
1¼ cups boiling water
1 cup sour cream
½ cup mayonnaise or salad dressing
2 medium avocados, peeled and cubed
½ small onion
1¼ tbsp. Spirulina

1 tbsp. lemon juice
½ tsp. vegetable salt (to taste)
1 head red leaf lettuce
orange sections/grapefruit sections
mayonnaise
cayenne or black pepper (optional)

1. Put gelatin in blender, add boiling water and blend with lid adjusted till gelatin has dissolved.
2. Add sour cream, mayonnaise, avocado, onion, Spirulina, lemon juice and salt to gelatin mix. This may have to be done in two batches, depending on size of blender.
3. Blend till smooth.
4. Pour into a 4½-5 cup decorative mold and chill until firm.
5. Unmold on lettuce.
6. Arrange orange and grapefruit sections around unmolded salad in a decorative manner.
7. Serve with added mayonnaise if desired. Some cayenne or black pepper may be added to the mayonnaise (optional).

Serves 6-8.

WALNUT AND AVOCADO SALAD

2-3 tbsp. lemon juice
3 ripe avocados
3 sweet crisp apples
3 oz. walnuts
3-5 tbsp. French dressing
1½ tbsp. Spirulina
1 clove garlic (optional)
seasoning

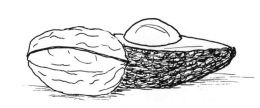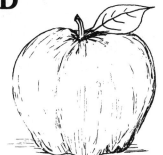

1. Put the lemon juice into a bowl.
2. Carefully cut avocados in half and remove the pits. Scrape the avocado flesh gently into the bowl without damaging the skins.
3. Mash with the lemon juice. (This prevents it from turning brown.)
4. Core the apples, chop them and the walnuts into small pieces and mix with the avocado pulp, French dressing, Spirulina, crushed garlic (if you wish) and a little seasoning.
5. Blend well and gently refill the avocado shells.
6. Place on bed of lettuce leaves.
7. Garnish with cherry tomato and parsley leaves.

Other garnishes could be sliced pepper and cucumber or sliced hard boiled eggs.

Serves 6.

SUMMER SALMON OR TUNA SALAD

7 oz. can tuna or salmon, undrained and
   flaked
2 stalks thinly sliced celery
3 green onions, finely sliced
1 tbsp. snipped fresh coriander leaves
   (available in specialty stores)

2 tsp. chili sauce
1 tsp. soy sauce
½ tsp. ginger powder
1 tbsp. Spirulina
2 avocados

1. Mix together all the above ingredients except the avocados. Refrigerate, covered, for at least 2 hours.
2. Cut avocados in half. Remove pits.
3. Fill cavity with salad and serve with garlic bread and a glass of iced cold Rosé.

Serves 4.

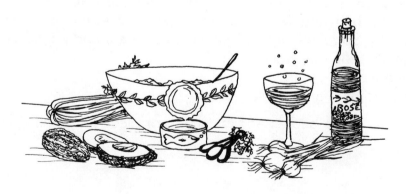

FRESH TOMATO/SPIRULINA ASPIC

Hits the spot on a hot summer afternoon.

4 medium tomatoes, peeled, seeded and cut
   in quarters
2 stalks celery, sliced
⅓ small onion
1 tbsp. Spirulina
2 tbsp. honey

2 tbsp. lemon juice
½ tsp. salt or to taste
½ tsp. celery salt
dash of hot pepper sauce (optional)
2 tbsp. agar agar flakes (available in health
   food stores)
¾ cup cold water

1. Blend tomatoes in blender until puréed.
2. Add celery, onion, Spirulina, honey, lemon juice, salt and hot pepper sauce.
3. Blend till vegetables are finely chopped.
4. In a small saucepan soften the agar agar flakes in cold water.
5. Place over low heat and stir till agar agar is dissolved.
6. Add to tomato/Spirulina mixture.
7. Turn into ring mold.
8. Chill till firm.
9. To serve, unmold, and if you wish, fill the center with peeled, cubed cucumber or peeled, cubed jicama or radishes. (Jicama is available in specialty or Mexican food stores.)

Serves 6.

GOTU KOLA MALLUNG SALAD

This dish is a must in every Ceylonese home.

*2 bunches Gotu Kola or watercress
½ fresh coconut, grated (you could use the unsweetened coconut available in health food stores)
1 tbsp. bonito flakes (optional—available in Japanese food stores)

¼ tsp. turmeric
½ tsp. salt or to taste
juice of lemon or lime
4 shallots, finely sliced, or green onions
1 green pepper, hot or mild according to taste, chopped fine
2 tsp. Spirulina

1. Wash watercress, discarding hard stems, and put the leaves in a bowl (the tender stems should be used as well).
2. Grate coconut and add the rest of the ingredients and mix very well.
3. Just before serving combine the coconut mixture with the watercress leaves and toss well.

Delicious served with a rice and curry meal. Full of iron and other goodies.

*We are using watercress here as it is more readily available than Gotu Kola. You may of course use other tender greens finely sliced, i.e., chard, carrot tops, beet tops, cabbage, etc.

Serves 4-6.

RADISH AND JICAMA SALAD

Jicama is available in specialty or Mexican food stores.

3 tbsp. Dijon mustard
1 tbsp. lemon juice
1 tbsp. white wine vinegar
¾ tsp. salt or to taste
1 garlic clove, crushed
1 tsp. dry mustard
¼-½ tsp. pepper

1 tbsp. Spirulina
½ cup vegetable oil
1½ cups finely sliced jicama (or sliced turnips)
1½ cups finely sliced radishes
6 green onions with tops, chopped
¼ cup fresh snipped parsley

1. Combine Dijon mustard, lemon juice, vinegar, salt, garlic, dry mustard, pepper and Spirulina in a small bowl.
2. Whisk in oil gradually.
3. Refrigerate, covered, for at least 3-4 hours for flavors to blend.
4. Combine radishes, jicama, onions and parsley in a large bowl.
5. Refrigerate, covered, 3-4 hours.
6. Toss radish/jicama mixture with mustard/Spirulina mixture just before serving.

Serves 6.

SPIRULINA AND WORLD HUNGER

"Now that the price is high and Spirulina in the USA is beginning to be a vitamin supplement, everybody is wanting to buy it and millionaires want to invest in it as a venture. Our "Possibility Thinker" realizes that one day we will produce thousands of tons of Spirulina; and then the prices will go cheaper and cheaper until poor hungry people can afford it. But it will probably get more expensive at the beginning—as long as there is a shortage and the cost of small-scale production is high. But even at today's prices it only works out at $1.00 per day because Spirulina is so concentrated and so nutritious that you only need a dollar's worth a day to stay alive. Try to get anyone in the USA or Japan to stay alive for $1.00 a day, or $365.00 a year!

—from THE SECRETS OF SPIRULINA, ed. by Christopher Hills

"The whole idea of harnessing the sun's light in Spirulina Plankton came to our founder, Dr. Christopher Hills, as a spiritual vision of bringing the deserts back to life and feeding the hungry, protein-starved world. He saw Spirulina as the God-given "manna from heaven", a medium of transmission that we can all use to undertake a new mission of working for cosmic Truth and helping the needy to tap abundant resources, all at the same time. Since 1967, as President of the Microalgae International Union, he has worked to create a tremendous networking which is now about to extend into refugee camps in Cambodia, Africa and Afghanistan to feed the hungry. Spirulina missionaries who can pay their own passage to refugee camps can get in touch with Dr. Hills. If they qualify he will see that some part of two million tablets of Spirulina reach the hungry through their hands."

University of the Trees Newsletter—February 1981

DRESSINGS

Tangy and nutritious energy boosters—we've included a wide variety here to satisfy the tastes of almost any dinner guest on your list. Make sure to whisk them well to remove any Spirulina lumps. The fruit dressings lend added variety and flavor.

BOILED DRESSING

Very, very good tossed with shredded cabbage.

3 egg yolks
⅓ cup cider vinegar
⅓ cup heavy cream
⅓ cup water
1 tbsp. butter
1 tbsp. honey
1 tsp. dry mustard
salt and pepper to taste
1 tbsp. Spirulina
½ tsp. sweet paprika

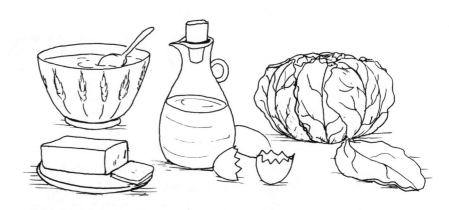

1. Combine first 7 ingredients in a heavy saucepan.
2. Simmer over low heat, stirring until thickened.
3. Add salt and pepper and whisk in Spirulina and paprika.

Makes about ¾ cup.

COCONUT CREAM DRESSING

1 cup coconut cream
½ lb. cottage cheese
salt and pepper to taste
2 tsp. honey
1 tbsp. Spirulina

Combine all the above ingredients together and mix well. (Blend if you have a blender.)

To make coconut cream if you cannot buy it already processed:

1. Break coconut in half.
2. In small batches, remove coconut meat from shell, cut in small pieces and put in blender.
3. Add ¾ cup warm water and blend till coconut and water are well combined.
4. Put in a sieve and squeeze out all the liquid.

Voilá—coconut milk or cream.

Makes 1½-2 cups.

SESAME DRESSING

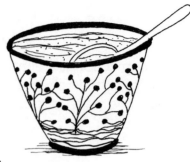

1 tbsp. Dijon mustard
1 tbsp. rice vinegar
1 tbsp. soy sauce
1 egg yolk
1 garlic clove, crushed and minced

1 tbsp. Spirulina
¼ cup vegetable oil
2 tbsp. sesame oil
1 tsp. lemon juice
salt and pepper to taste

1. Combine in a bowl mustard, vinegar, soy sauce, egg yolk and garlic clove.
2. Add Spirulina.
3. Add to the above mixture vegetable oil and sesame oil, pouring in a stream and whisking all the time.
4. Stir in lemon juice, salt and pepper.
5. Toss dressing with toasted sesame seeds and salad greens or meat and chicken salad.

Makes ¾ cup.

YOGURT DRESSING

Good on lunchtime salad, especially in the summer.

3 tbsp. orange juice
2 tbsp. honey
1 tbsp. lemon juice
½ tbsp. Spirulina
1 tbsp. fresh chopped mint (or ½ tbsp. dried)
1 cup natural yogurt

1. Combine orange juice, honey, lemon juice, Spirulina and mint.
2. Whisk in natural yogurt.
3. Toss the dressing with orange sections and seedless grapes.

Makes about 1⅓ cups.

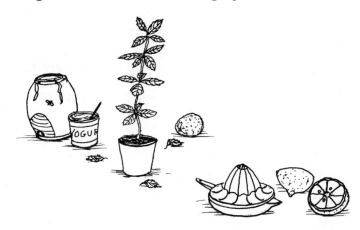

ORANGE AND NUT DRESSING

Rich and crunchy.

6 tbsp. orange juice
1½ tbsp. honey
¼-½ tsp. dry mustard (to taste)
salt and pepper to taste
4 tbsp. oil
3 tbsp. chopped walnuts
1 tbsp. Spirulina

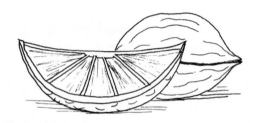

1. Blend orange juice, honey, seasoning and Spirulina.
2. Add oil and nuts.
3. Garnish with crumbled bacon bits or diced water chestnuts.

Delicious on a salad of tender young carrot tops, beet tops or shredded chicory and onion leaves.

Makes about ¾ cup.

SIBYL'S DRESSING

Tomato sweet/sour.

1 cup safflower oil
⅓ cup vinegar
3 tbsp. tomato sauce
1 heaping tbsp. Spirulina
1 tsp. mustard

¼ tsp. oregano
⅛ tsp. salt
dash cayenne
1 tbsp. tamari
1 tsp. honey

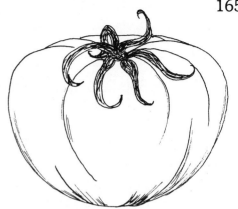

Blend together all ingredients.

TOMATO DRESSING WITH SPIRULINA

Delicious with seafood salads.

1 cup tomato, peeled, seeded and chopped
¼ cup minced onion
1 tbsp. minced fresh parsley
2 tbsp. minced basil

½ tsp. honey
1 tbsp. Spirulina
salt and pepper to taste
½ cup French dressing (made with Dijon mustard)

1. Combine in a bowl the tomato, onion, parsley, basil, honey, Spirulina, salt and pepper.
2. Add French dressing in a stream, whisking.

Makes about 2 cups.

PAM'S DRESSING

Spirulina/olive oil.

Mix Spirulina to taste into olive oil with some miso and a mild vinegar (like Japanese vinegar) or basil vinegar. Olive oil is the only oil thick enough to hold the Spirulina in suspension.

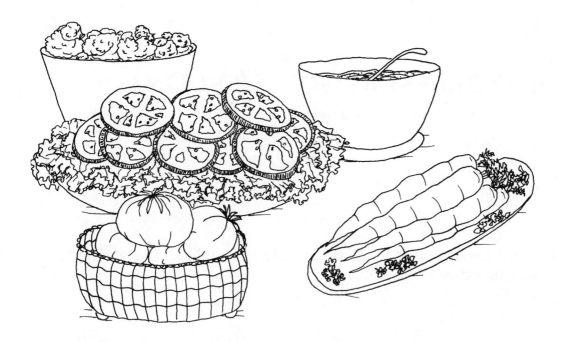

DESSERTS

Would that we could do away with desserts entirely as far as our health and waistlines go. But the will is weak and our children demanding so there is often a call for a tasty sweetie at the end of a meal. We do not use sugar in this book so you'll find all the desserts sweetened with honey. Spirulina recipes from fruit dishes to cookies to ice cream give you a wide range to choose from to complement any meal.

BANANA CREAM HAWAIIAN

An extra zip with a touch of rum.

2 cups mashed bananas
¼ cup honey or to taste
⅛ tsp. salt
½ cup pineapple juice

2 tbsp. rum
1 tsp. powdered ginger
½ tbsp. Spirulina
1 cup heavy cream (whipping)
sesame seeds or toasted coconut (optional)

1. Mix together the bananas, honey, salt, pineapple juice, lemon juice, rum, ginger and Spirulina.
2. Whip the cream till stiff, fold into the banana mixture and turn into a freezing tray.
3. Freeze in the freezer compartment of the refrigerator with control set at coldest point or in a freezer until the edges are mushy.
4. Turn into a bowl and beat until frothy.
5. Return to tray and freeze until set.

As an optional addition I have found toasted sesame seeds quite delicious with this combination. Toasted coconut may also be used as a topping.

Serves 6-8.

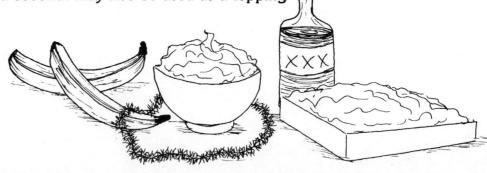

COCONUT PUDDING

⅔ cup cornstarch
½ cup honey (or to taste)
1 qt. milk or a mixture of milk and half and half
pinch of salt
15½ oz. can Coconut Cream (available from liquor section of supermarket)
1 tbsp. Spirulina
4 oz. pistachio nuts, chopped, or nuts of your choice
½ cup flaked coconut

1. Mix cornstarch and honey in a saucepan.
2. Gradually stir in the milk, salt and Coconut Cream.
3. Cook over low heat, stirring steadily, until thickened.
4. Whisk in the Spirulina and stir in the chopped nuts.
5. Pour into a buttered pan and sprinkle with coconut.
6. Chill.
7. Cut into squares.

The pistachio nuts give a delicious and uncommon flavor. You may also lightly toast the coconut before sprinkling on the pudding. This recipe has gotten raves every time I've served it.

Serves 10-15.

COCONUT ICE CREAM

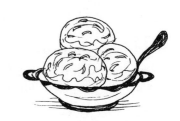

2 tbsp. vanilla
1 tbsp. arrowroot
1½ cups milk (coconut if preferred)
4 egg yolks
½ cup honey
pinch of sea salt
2½ cups unsweetened natural shredded coconut (available in health food stores)
2½ cups whipping cream
3 tbsp. Spirulina

1. In top of double boiler mix together vanilla, arrowroot and milk.
2. Cook for 5 minutes.
3. Beat egg yolks lightly with honey and salt.
4. Add to hot vanilla mixture.
5. Cook, stirring constantly, until thickened.
6. Cool.
7. Add coconut, heavy cream and Spirulina to the mixture.
8. Churn freeze in an electric ice cream maker.

The taste of coconut in this mixture is quite delicious. You may try for variation to top it with crushed pineapple.

Serves 6.

AVOCADO DELIGHT

2 med. ripe avocados
5 tbsp. lime or lemon juice
⅔ cup honey
1 cup natural raspberry preserves
6 tbsp. finely chopped preserved ginger
    (available in Chinese grocery)
pinch of salt
1 tbsp. Spirulina
2 cups whipping cream
⅔ cup light cream (half and half)

1. Cut avocados in half, peel and purée in an electric blender or food mill.
2. Combine avocado purée with lime juice, honey, raspberry preserves, ginger and salt.
3. Blend until smooth.
4. Add Spirulina and blend well.
5. Whip cream lightly and fold into avocado mixture.
6. Chill in freezer compartment of refrigerator.
7. Top with light cream before serving.

Serves 4.

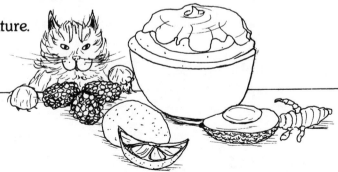

SPIRULINA FRUIT FANTASIA

A yummy party treat.

⅓ cup honey
6 tbsp. crushed pineapple
1 mashed banana
½ cup chopped strawberries
2 oranges, peeled and diced

1 tbsp. lemon juice
1 pkg. unflavored gelatin
¼ cup cold water
1½ cups whipping cream
½ cup cashew nuts, slightly roasted
1½ tbsp. Spirulina

1. Combine honey, pineapple, banana, strawberries, oranges and lemon juice.
2. Blend until smooth.
3. Soften gelatin in water for 5 minutes.
4. Heat gelatin and water mixture and stir until dissolved.
5. Beat heavy cream until lightly whipped.
6. Add dissolved gelatin, cashew nuts, whipped cream and Spirulina to the fruit mixture.
7. Churn freeze in electric ice cream maker.

Served with a nut cream sauce this is delicious and appealing.

Simple Nut Cream Sauce:
1 cup cashew nut butter
½ cup milk.

   Mix well.

Serves 4.

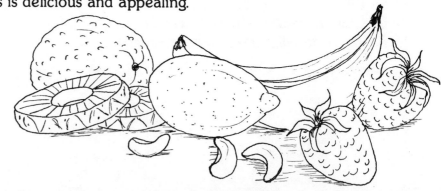

SPIRULINA DROP COOKIES

½ cup oil
1 cup maple syrup
1 cup flour
½ tsp. baking soda
1 tbsp. (or more) Spirulina
1 cup coconut
1 cup roasted peanuts
1 cup raisins
1 cup sunflower seeds
1 cup carob chips (optional)

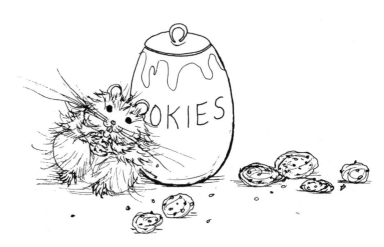

1. Mix oil and syrup.
2. Add flour, soda, Spirulina, coconut.
3. Mix well.
4. Add remaining ingredients and mix well.
5. Drop on greased cookie sheets and bake at 350° for 15-20 minutes.

Makes 30-40.

MAGIC PUFFS

Mincemeat/Spirulina triangles.

Filling:
1 lb. jar mincemeat or 1 pkg. condensed mincemeat
2 tbsp. Spirulina

Combine together and set aside.

Cream:
2 cups milk
2 in. piece lemon peel
6 egg yolks
½ cup honey or to taste
¼ cup flour
2 tbsp. Spirulina

1. In a small saucepan scald the milk with lemon peel.
2. In a bowl beat the egg yolks with the honey and flour until the mixture is light and lemon-colored.
3. Add the milk in a stream, stirring.
4. Transfer the mixture to a saucepan and cook it over moderate heat, stirring constantly for 5 minutes or until it is thick.
5. Discard the lemon peel and chill the cream, covered, for at least 1 hour in refrigerator.

Pastry:

2 cups flour
¾ stick butter or margarine (cut into bits)
1 tsp. each salt and ground anise seed
2 egg yolks
¼ cup sour cream
¼ cup medium dry sherry

1. In another bowl blend the flour, butter, salt and anise until the mixture resembles meal.
2. In a small bowl beat the egg yolks with the sour cream and sherry.
3. Stir the mixture into the flour and stir until it is well combined.
4. Form the dough into a ball and chill it, wrapped in wax paper for about 1 hour.
5. Halve the dough, roll out each half ⅛" thick on a floured surface.
6. Cut into 5 inch squares with a cutter.
7. Place 1 teaspoonful of mincemeat/Spirulina mixture, which has been well combined, in center of pastry square and top with ½-¾ tablespoon pastry cream.
8. Fold the squares diagonally to form triangles and pinch the edges together.
9. In a deep fryer fry the pastries, about 4-5 at a time, in about 3 inches hot vegetable oil, turning them frequently for 4 minutes, or bake them at 350° till golden brown—10-15 minutes.
10. Transfer the pastries as they are done to paper towels to drain.
11. Sprinkle with brown sugar if you wish.

Makes 24 pastries of delectable magic.

SPIRULINA FRUIT AND NUT CAKES

2 cups dried apricots
2 cups dates
1 cup dried pears
1 cup raisins

1 cup peanuts, sunflower seeds or almonds
3 tbsp. Spirulina
toasted coconut
pinch of cinnamon (optional)
vanilla (up to 1 tsp.)

1. Chop all the fruit in food processor or mince.
2. Chop nuts coarsely and mix in well with fruit and Spirulina.
3. Form into small cakes and roll in toasted coconut. (If too dry, moisten with vanilla.)

Makes 1 dozen cakes.

GOLDEN DELICIOUS SPIRULINASAUCE

5 large apples
¼ cup almonds
½ tsp. lemon juice

¼ tsp. cinnamon (to taste)
shake of nutmeg and ginger
water to cover
1-1½ tbsp. Spirulina

1. Quarter and remove core from apples.
2. Cut into pieces and simmer with remaining ingredients (except Spirulina) until tender.
3. Put in blender, add Spirulina and blend until smooth.
4. Serve in dessert cups with slices of warm buttered gingerbread.

Serves 6.

GOURMET FASTING

Fasting needn't be a misery. We can leave behind the days of enduring water, or zucchini broth, or lemon juice and honey in order to cleanse and rejuvenate. Spirulina is nature's perfect gift for those of us interested in detoxifying, eliminating, and giving our systems a rest while at the same time staying properly nourished and well fueled enough to work.

There are as many ways to fast with Spirulina as there are liquids to mix it with. Apple juice and Spirulina. Carrot juice and Spirulina (a rich one). Spirulina with fresh squeezed orange juice. V-8 or tomato juice, Spirulina, and a dash of Tabasco (olé!). Spirulina blends well with papaya juice, and is especially delicious with pineapple-coconut juice, or plain pineapple juice.

The following recipes have been tried and tested and proven to be our favorites here at the University of the Trees community. In fact, when we're not fasting they still turn up on the breakfast or lunch table (or in a thermos if we're traveling) because they're fast, they're quick energy, they're filling, and most important they leave us with that light feeling of having just done something really good for our bodies.

Spirulina with Apple Juice

Try heating it, adding a dash of cinnamon and a teaspoon of nutritional yeast. The amount of Spirulina will vary to taste.

Sparkling Apple Cider

⅔ cup apple juice
⅓ cup sparkling water
1 tsp. or more of Spirulina

This bubbler is a wonderful summer drink.

Spirulina—Miso Combinations

Pour into a blender 1½ cups of water (enough for one serving). Add a generous spoonful of miso. Blend. Add generous spoonful of Spirulina—at least one teaspoonful. Blend again. Heat gently but do not boil. This is the basic recipe. Double or triple if desired. Our favorite variations are as follows:

1. Add a generous spoonful of tahini (sesame butter). Optional seasonings—flavor with curry, or a dash of sherry, or some mustard. Tahini when blended is easy to digest, and the calcium content is a perfect complement to the Spirulina.
2. Add tahini, and other nut butters, like roasted almond butter, raw cashew butter, or peanut butter.
3. Add cayenne to warm you on cold winter mornings!
4. Add nutritional yeast.

My current favorite is a blend of V-8 juice, miso, tahini, roasted almond butter, yeast, Spirulina and cayenne. It's outrageously delicious. If you're not fasting, try it for lunch with crackers. I also enjoy soaking seaweed (arame, hiziki, wakame or kombu) beforehand and adding it to my soups. Kind of like noodles, and kids like them too.

Miso Tahini Spirulina Soup

Here's Roger's version:

6 cups water
4 cloves garlic
2 tbsp. tahini

4 tbsp. miso
5 tbsp. Spirulina
1 tsp. curry
black pepper to taste

This is a wonderful broth for fasting. For regular meals add diced tofu or whatever vegetables are on hand. Green onions are nice, too.

These basic ingredients can be combined in an infinite number of ways to suit your taste. Our bodies appreciate the rest from digesting solid foods, and our blood cells appreciate the chlorophyll to help with cleansing and detoxifying. Fasting becomes a creative experience that leaves you fulfilled and filled full.

And finally the drink that Debbie swears by every morning:

Debbie's Delight

1 cup warm water
4 tsp. lactobacillus Bifidus powder
2 tsp. Spirulina

Debbie says, "Purchase Bifidus (Eugalen Topfer Forte is one available brand name) at a health food store. It's excellent for building and maintaining the intestinal flora and aids digestion. Combined with Spirulina, it makes a perfect breakfast."

Let us hear from you. Share your own unique successes with recipes and with fasting, and join the growing number of people who eat Light!

Nancy London

INDEX

MORE . . . on Spirulina!

REJUVENATING THE BODY Through Fasting With Spirulina Plankton, by Christopher Hills, Ph.D., D.Sc.
The world's newest "super" food has actually been known to the Aztec and African cultures for centuries. In Japan it is a staple part of the diet and is even fed to prize-winning fish. An 85-year-old man has lived on nothing else for the past 15 years. What is it? Spirulina Plankton, the total food for health, rejuvenation and survival. *Rejuvenating the Body* describes practical uses for Spirulina, the highest form of natural vegetable protein available on this planet. Thousands of people are discovering the benefits of this remarkable food and nutritional supplement. *Rejuvenating the Body* contains a complete, easy-to-follow program to cleanse our bodies and bring back vigor and the blush of health.
153,000 copies of this book are now in print. Illustrated, 64 pp., $2.50.

THE SECRETS OF SPIRULINA: Medical Discoveries of Japanese Doctors, Edited by Dr. Christopher Hills. Japanese editor, Dr. Naoharu Fujii, M.D.
This is the first book published in the West documenting the medical benefits of Spirulina researched in Japan. Spirulina plankton is the amazing form of algae that is the most complete food product on the planet. Fifteen Japanese medical doctors and researchers collaborated to produce this book, now translated into English for the first time. Their unanimous conclusion: *Spirulina is not only a complete food for total health and is quickly becoming the superior vitamin supplement, but it is also a remarkable aid in the treatment of various chronic diseases such as diabetes, hepatitis, glaucoma.* 200 pp., $6.95.
NOTE: In the USA no medical claims can be made, due to FDA regulations.

FOOD FROM SUNLIGHT, by Christopher Hills and Hiroshi Nakamura.
Of all the problems facing our planet hunger is one of the most perplexing and saddening. Starvation is a reality for perhaps two-thirds of the earth's people, and each day we seem to hear of famine hitting yet another part of the globe. At last there is a solution: microalgae. *Food From Sunlight* tells every aspect of its potential to feed the world: how to grow algae, facts and figures about the amazing nutritional benefits of Chlorella and Spirulina, two superior strains, and how to bring our deserts and exhausted lands back into productive use. Algae is an excellent source of energy and some strains even thrive on pollution. Every survivalist will want to get his hands on this invaluable book. Well illustrated, 384 pp., $14.95.

Include $1.00 postage and handling per book. All prices subject to change without notice.

WHAT IS UNIVERSITY OF THE TREES?

Most people who do not live with us from day to day only have contact with us through our worldly activities—our books, tapes, tools, or nutritional foods—because our spiritual mission is definitely low profile. There are so many sensation-hunters in the spiritual supermarket that we prefer to communicate our teachings to the smaller circle of those who have long-term staying power and avoid the fanatics or the gullibility of those who make important the outward trappings—changes of clothes, changes of names, public display or religious show biz and other superficial ego mechanisms.

So much goes on here daily at University of the Trees in a very intense manifestation that we may sometimes forget our main purpose which is to draw you closer to our community vibration. Our community is not for those who need the support of others as a crutch but for those who use it as a means of becoming more selfless and as an instrument for serving the world more effectively than they could as a single individual. Our community is a veritable hot house for growth and most people who came here two or three or five years ago are now utterly different than when they came. They are strong, confident and totally effective! With such people we can tackle problems which are not even looked at by schools, politicians and group leaders, yet without new solutions all the present schemes for salvation are worthless. This also applies in the religious domain where the ego is hardly tackled and relationships with God are even touted by many as self-righteous ego food rather than a humbling experience. Despite all the preaching, people don't really change deeply except by what humbles them. That is a sobering thought!

You are always invited to join the spiritual side of our work as well as participate in our other endeavors, like our first steps to feed the world with Spirulina or bring mankind to understand the nature of his own consciousness with our books. The spiritual side is the most important and is beyond words or promotional protestations. Our whole life is a feeling of closeness and being part of an ongoing spiritual/economic enterprise which is linked with the cosmic will. All the steps are provided already by an infinite intelligence and it is our part to participate in the excitement of discovering them for the future and for history.

Christopher Hills

HOW TO GET SPIRULINA

The FDA has not approved Spirulina as a food, but they do allow it to be sold as a nutritional supplement. Spirulina has been approved by the Japanese equivalent of the FDA and by the FDA in Mexico.

Potentized Spirulina, as used in these recipes and approved by Dr. Hills, can be obtained from your local health food store under the label of Aquaculture Nutrition Products. It is also available from distributors of Light Force Spirulina Company. Be sure that any Spirulina you purchase has no artificial additives or fillers and is potentized, as this has been found to make a considerable difference.

If you cannot obtain supplies in your area write to the publishers of this book.